arthritis

and how to live with it

GW00597454

arthritis

and **how** to **live** with it

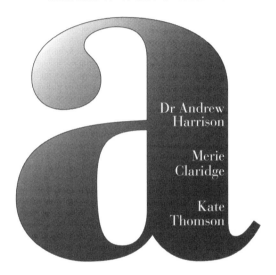

Dr Andrew
Harrison

Merie
Claridge

Kate
Thomson

RANDOM HOUSE
NEW ZEALAND

The publisher would like to thank Victor Marks for his tireless effort and contribution to the Lifecare Series.

Other titles in the Lifecare Series include:
Cancer — and how to live with it; Denise Robbins
Diabetes — and how to live with it; Louise Farmer, Sue Pearson, Amber Strong
Food matters — a guide to healthy eating and supplements; Suzi Penny
Heart disease — and how to live with it; Victor Marks, Dr Monica Lewis, Dr Gerald Lewis
Postnatal moods — emotional changes following birth; Gillian White
Pregnancy — a guide to healthy pregnancy in New Zealand; Ann Noseworthy, Jacques Rousseau
Toxic chemicals and you; Suzi Penny, Stephen Bell
Asthma — and how to live with it; Dr Shaun Holt, Robyn Ingleton, Kim van Griensven

A catalogue record for this book is available from the National Library of New Zealand

A RANDOM HOUSE BOOK
published by
Random House New Zealand
18 Poland Road, Glenfield, Auckland, New Zealand

www.randomhouse.co.nz

First published 2006

© 2006 Massey University Institute of Food, Nutrition and Human Health, New Zealand

ISBN-13: 978 1 86941 777 2
ISBN-10: 1 86941 777 1

Series coordinator: Victor Marks
Cover design: Katy Yiakmis
Design: Kate Greenaway
Printed in Australia by Griffin Press

Dedication

We would like to dedicate this book to three very special groups of people:

Firstly, the team at Arthritis New Zealand; the educators, support staff, the volunteers, members and donors, whose invaluable contribution ensures that people in New Zealand with arthritis have access to all the services that enable them to maximise the quality of their lives both at home and in the community.

Secondly, the rheumatology health professionals who, even though in scant supply, willingly commit additional unpaid hours to speak at seminars, conferences and to provide lobbying support for access to better treatment and medicines for their patients.

Finally and most importantly, all New Zealanders with arthritis, whose courage and positive attitude are an inspiration to us all.

Acknowledgements

We gratefully acknowledge the contribution of Mr Chris Bossley, orthopaedic surgeon, who wrote the chapter on surgery.

And to Victor Marks whose insights and turns of phrase converted our technical shorthand into something that a patient might understand, thank you.

Contents

Part two Types of arthritis

Part three Living with arthritis

Introduction

Thanks to the research that's been done throughout the world over the past few years, we now know much more about arthritis than ever before. Though we can't yet cure it we've learned how to handle it so that with the correct management, it's possible for people with arthritis to live full and fulfilling lives.

In this book we'll take a look at what's been learned and how we can best use this knowledge to improve the quality of our lives and the satisfaction there is to be found in living them. In plain everyday language we'll tell you about arthritis as an illness — how you can best manage it, slow down its progression, and live a comfortable satisfied life.

In part one we'll concentrate on the more clinical side of arthritis. This will include:

- The disease itself, the many forms it can take and the signs and symptoms you're likely to experience
- How to build a relationship with the health professionals you'll most probably come across, e.g. rheumatologist, rheumatology nurse, occupational therapist and physiotherapist
- The tests you'll have, what the doctor will ask you, and what you should have ready to reply
- Pain management — how to work your way through the maze of medications available and finding the best ones for you
- Complementary therapies — though we live in the Western world and our first call for treatment is on conventional Western medicine, more and more of us are seeking to augment our care by also trying such treatments

Part two is where we take a much closer look at some of the different forms of arthritis.

In part three we'll get a little more personal and look at ways to manage your arthritis and how you can draw up a lifestyle self-management plan. This will include:

- The what? where? why? and how? of exercise with a few ideas that will do you the world of good
- How healthy eating can be a great tonic for both body and mind
- The relationship between our bodies and our minds and how one can affect the other
- The techniques that will help reduce any anxiety or stress you may be feeling

To finish off there are some appendices which we hope you will find useful.

In writing this book our aim has been to bring you the most up-to-date information on arthritis and the current treatments that are available. It's not meant to be read through from cover to cover as you would a novel, but rather it's a book to be dipped into to answer questions you may have regarding your own particular condition.

Finally, as you read through the various sections that interest you, keep in mind the three words that Arthritis New Zealand uses as its battle cry — DISCOVER YOU CAN.

Why this book needed to be written

In New Zealand today we are privileged to be able to enjoy a comfortable standard of living despite the fact that Australians earn more than us. Thankfully, we can argue that we enjoy a quality of life here that's not known in many other countries.

Well . . . for some of us that's very true. Unfortunately, however, many people who have arthritis feel disadvantaged and that their condition is prohibiting them from being able to enjoy the benefits of this wonderful country we call home.

This need not be so!

Although we can't yet cure arthritis, we can learn how to handle it — with the correct management it's possible for people with arthritis to live full and satisfying lives.

That is why this book has been written: to present an overview of arthritis and, in simple everyday language, explain how, by recognising the disease early enough and using the knowledge gained from scientific research, someone with arthritis can manage their condition, slow down its progress and enjoy the benefits this country has to offer.

The authors are New Zealanders who each bring a different perspective to the subject:

- Andrew Harrison, MB, ChB, FRACP, PhD is a rheumatologist, a specialist who understands the diseases
- Merie Claridge is specialist rheumatology nurse with the Hutt Valley District Health Board, who understands and deals with the everyday problems of people with arthritis
- Kate Thomson, President, Arthritis New Zealand, is a patient who lives with arthritis every day of her life

These three people have brought together their experience and knowledge to help you and your family understand the nature of the different types of arthritis, explain who's there to help you and suggest ways you can help yourself.

Some facts and figures

At the last count there were over 520,000 people in New Zealand living with arthritis — that's more than the population of Wellington, Lower Hutt, Upper Hutt, Porirua and Kapiti combined, and:

- Over half are female (57.6 per cent) — that's more than the combined populations of Otago and Southland
- Over half are of working age (16–65)
- 9.2 per cent are of Maori descent — that's more than the entire population of the Waikato region

The total financial cost of arthritis in New Zealand in 2005 was estimated to be $2.35 billion. This includes:

- 25,440 New Zealanders who did not work in 2005 because of arthritis — costing an estimated $1 billion in lost productivity
- Temporary absences from work due to arthritis — costing an estimated $18 million in lost productivity

Part one

About arthritis

True or false?

Being overweight heightens the risk of getting arthritis.
True
This is especially true for osteoarthritis.

All people with arthritis will at some time need surgery.
False
Most people with arthritis will never need surgery.

If my anti-inflammatory medication is not working I can combine
it with any over-the-counter pain reliever.
False
Some over-the-counter pain relievers are anti-inflammatory
drugs themselves; for example, Nurofen. Always ask your
pharmacist or doctor first.

Chapter 1

What is arthritis?

Arthritis comes from two Greek words, *arthron* (joint) and *itis* (inflammation), and literally means inflamed joint, though the term is nowadays more likely to be used to indicate any disorder of the joints. While in the past many people referred to the disease as *rheumatism*, the current term, and the one we use in this book, is arthritis.

While the origin of the word arthritis is from the Greek, the disease had been around for quite some time before that great civilisation. Archaeologists examining dinosaur bones have found evidence indicating that the disease existed 85,000,000 years ago. The first evidence that humans were subject to the disease comes from around 30,000 years ago with arthritis found in the bones of a prehistoric Neanderthal man. Today the disease is found in all corners of the world and is particularly, but not exclusively, a disease we experience as we get older.

Arthritis through the ages

c. 85,000,000 BC: Dinosaur bones show that many of them had osteoarthritis in their ankles.

c. 30,000–28,000 BC: Remains of Neanderthal man show that many of them had secondary osteoarthritis.

c. 4500 BC: The earliest known appearance of rheumatoid arthritis is found in the bones of North American Indians.

c. 2590 BC: The mummified bodies of the great Kings of Egypt and their lowly servants give us early proof that arthritis draws no distinction between the rich and the poor.

c. 500 BC: Man uses the salicin (found in ground willow bark) to reduce aches and pains.

c. 400 BC: Hippocrates, the father of modern medicine, recognises gout and other joint ailments.

c. 40 BC: The great Roman Emperor, Julius Caesar, is known to have had arthritis.

c. AD 300: In Rome, citizens with severe arthritis are exempt from taxation.

1600: The French physician Guillame Baillou (1538–1616) introduces the idea of rheumatism as a systemic, musculoskeletal condition.

1754: Scleroderma is first identified.

1800: A Parisian doctor makes the first documentation of what later becomes known as rheumatoid arthritis.

1845: Viennese pathologist Ferdinand von Hebra describes what later becomes known as lupus.

1851: French physician Pierre Louis Alphee Cazenave applies the term *lupus erythematosus* to a skin disorder.

1858: The term *rheumatoid arthritis* is coined by British physician A.B. Garrod.

1886: The term *osteoarthritis* is coined by British physician John K. Spender.

1897: George F. Still reports the first mention of juvenile rheumatoid arthritis.

1897: Aspirin (synthetic salicin) is created by German chemist Felix Hoffman. It is manufactured commercially by Bayer and Co., 2500 years after the discovery of the benefits of ground willow bark to reduce aches and pains.

1933: Henrik Sjögren, a Swedish ophthalmologist, gives his name to *Sjögren's syndrome*.

1949: Philip Hench, MD, and Edward Kendall, PhD, use cortisone for the first time to treat rheumatoid arthritis.

Types of arthritis

The word 'arthritis' is used as an umbrella term for a number of diseases that each have their own cause, symptoms and treatment. While each has its own identity we divide them into two categories:

Non-inflammatory arthritis: Also known as *osteoarthritis*, this is a form of arthritis that, though mainly a result of the aging process, can also result from factors such as genes and trauma. Just as motor cars suffer wear and tear, so too do we. We discuss osteoarthritis in more detail in Chapter 5, page 49.

Inflammatory arthritis: This includes all other types of arthritis that are not caused by aging or trauma, but are the result of an immune response within the body. The most common example is rheumatoid arthritis and we'll take a closer look at this in Chapter 6, page 53.

While distinctly different, both categories have some things in common, which include:

- Affecting some part of a joint
- Causing pain and possibly limiting movement
- The likelihood of some swelling

As all the conditions affect one or other of the joints, let's first of all take a look at how the human body is put together, the role of the joints, and how we use them in our everyday lives.

The human body

Your skeleton and the muscles that connect more than 200 bones and 150 joints that make up your body give you the flexibility and freedom to sit, walk, talk, run and do all those fun things that humans do.

Synovial joints

The most common joints in your body, synovial joints, allow you to bend, turn and reach up or down. When they're all working together you're able to play sport or dance to a merry tune or two. Here's how they work:

- Joints are the sophisticated hinges that join bones together and give your body flexibility
- Joints are held together by *ligaments*
- Joints are controlled by *tendons*, which join the muscles to bone
- To prevent friction, each joint has a smooth layer of *cartilage* lining the surface of each bone where they make

contact, which is lubricated by a tiny amount of slippery liquid, *synovial fluid*, that is held in a special lining (the *synovial membrane* or *synovium*)

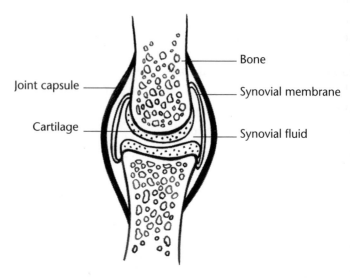

Joint capsule

Cartilage

Bone

Synovial membrane

Synovial fluid

A healthy joint showing the relationship between the synovial membrane and fluid, the cartilage, the joint capsule and the bone.

Types of synovial joints

Given the variety of activities we perform every day it's not surprising that we have a range of different joints that allow us to get through the everyday chores of living. Let's look at some of the more common ones:

Hinge joints: They work just like the hinge of a door, opening one way only. We have them in our fingers, elbows and knees.

Saddle joints: Similar to the hinge joint, but these can also move side to side. Have a look at your wrist and thumb.

Gliding joints: Your backbone is made up of bones with flat surfaces that glide over each other.

Ball-and-socket joints: The Rolls Royce of joints, they'll give you movement up or down, backwards or forwards, even around in circles. You'll find them in your hips and shoulders.

What causes arthritis?

When the joint systems are working properly, they allow us to move gracefully and seemingly without effort or even conscious thought. But when a joint is damaged or inflamed, we get mechanical breakdown that affects the joint's function, which in time can cause a weakening of its controlling muscles. And, of course, a great deal of pain.

So what causes this breakdown?

Unfortunately there isn't one simple answer that we can offer; rather we must look at a number of factors, each having its own influence depending on the type of arthritis we're considering. Here are the main contributing factors:

Heredity: In general, your genetic susceptibility can be influenced by a number of environmental and physical factors such as infection, trauma and obesity.

Age: Just as your hair becomes grey and your eyes begin to fail you, so too will your bones and joints suffer the effects of time.

Infection: Viruses, bacteria and fungi can be triggers that set off some forms of arthritis, particularly *infectious arthritis*.

Injury (trauma): If you suffer an injury to one of your joints the odds are that you could well develop problems with that joint in the future.

Overuse: If you are repeatedly pushing joints to their limit the chances are that you could develop arthritis in the future.

Other factors that can contribute to the development of the disease are:

- Obesity (which places excessive weight on joints)
- Problems with the immune system
- An influx of white blood cells that attack the joint lining

!! *A flare is when your signs and symptoms suddenly become worse. When this happens you need to immediately make an appointment with your GP, rheumatologist or rheumatology nurse so that it can be quickly brought under control. The longer a flare is left untreated, the harder it is to treat effectively.*

Signs and symptoms

The first indication most people get that all isn't as it should be is a developing awareness of some stiffness in a hip or knee, or perhaps they find their fingers aren't quite as nimble as they used to be. Also, they'll almost certainly notice some degree of pain in the affected joint(s).

Another indicator may be that there is some restriction in the range of movements they're used to enjoying.

Swelling can sometimes indicate the presence of arthritis, although swelling also occurs in other situations such as swollen ankles, which can result from heart, kidney or liver problems.

Some forms of arthritis are associated with symptoms that develop outside the joints; for example, *lupus* (a form of arthritis) shows itself by fever, hair loss or a rash brought on by exposure to sunlight. Another form of arthritis, *Sjogren's syndrome*, is characterised by dryness of the mouth and eyes. (See Chapter 8, page 62.)

!! Arthritis is not an easy condition to diagnose, so just because you feel stiff or a couple of joints hurt a little, it doesn't necessarily mean you have the disease.

See your doctor who, if he suspects a problem, will refer you to a specialist.

A final word

As you're reading this we assume that either you have, or you suspect you have, arthritis, or perhaps you're close to someone who has the disease. We further assume that you're seeking information so that you can understand this seemingly crippling disease and find out what can be done about it.

If this is the case, may we offer you the following advice: Don't panic!

Modern medicine has come a long way in the last few years, and although we can't yet cure arthritis we can certainly do much to control it. In many cases it is now possible to reverse some of the symptoms. Medications have improved and we now know and understand how individuals themselves can support their medical treatment by making changes in their lifestyle and adopting a positive mental attitude.

Chapter 2

Your friend — the doctor

Note: To avoid confusion we will refer to your doctor as a male 'him' rather than adopting the clumsy expression of 'him/her' or 'her/him'.

You've felt a few squeaks and twinges in the body, your knees might be giving you a bit of trouble and as for getting in and out of your chair, well, you'd be better off staying where you are but for the shopping you have to do and, goodness knows, the garden won't weed itself, now will it! Perhaps the symptoms are somewhat more focused. For example:

- You're finding that your joint pain is interfering with your everyday life
- The pain is lasting for more than a week
- Your sleep is being affected

If any of this rings a bell then it could well be time for you to go and have a chat with your doctor. The chances are you've been with the same GP for a number of years and he'll probably have a good knowledge of your medical history. This is important because the more information the doctor has, the better and quicker he can make a diagnosis of exactly what is wrong and the best way for it to be treated.

Determining if you have arthritis is not always an easy matter: the diagnosis in some cases may be immediately clear, but in others it could take weeks or even months to follow up clues and have all the necessary tests.

Preparing to see your doctor

One way you can help your doctor is to be as clear as you can about your symptoms and how they're affecting you. So, before going to the surgery give some thoughts to the following questions — as we all tend to fumble around a bit at the doctors. You may find it useful to write down your responses and take them with you.

Describing your symptoms

There are a number of questions your doctor will ask:

- When did the symptoms start?
- Which areas of your body are affected?
- Is there pain, swelling or stiffness?
- If you are experiencing pain, is it an ache, a burning sensation or a throb?
- How would you describe your pain on a scale of 1–10?
- Are the symptoms better after rest and made worse by activity?
- Are the symptoms worse after rest and then eased by movement?
- What is the impact on your daily life?
- Have other symptoms developed around the same time? For example:

  — Fever, sweats, reduced appetite, weight loss, fatigue

  — Rash, dryness of the eyes or mouth, circulation problems in your fingers or toes

  — Breathing problems and nerve symptoms, such as numbness or weakness

  — Diarrhoea or urinary problems

- What makes the symptoms better?
- What makes the symptoms worse?
- What other medical conditions do you have or have you had in the past?
- Are you taking any medication for another condition?

  (If you are it's a good idea to take it with you when you go to the doctor, including supplements.)

- Is there a family history of arthritis? (If you don't know, can you find out? If so, what type?)
- Is there a family history of *psoriasis* or *inflammatory bowel disease*?
- Have you had any recent injuries?
- To complete the picture your doctor will also want to be brought up to date about your domestic circumstances: If you work, what type of work do you do? Do you smoke? How much alcohol do you drink? Do you enjoy a healthy diet?

Having asked all his questions the doctor will physically examine you from head to toe paying particular attention to the joints in the area that's giving you pain or discomfort. Don't be surprised if he examines your other joints as this gives him a total picture and perhaps some vital clues as to the nature of the problem.

Some questions for your doctor

While your doctor is asking you all his questions you're sure to be worried about what he's going to find and you'll probably have plenty of questions of your own to ask him. He'll be well aware of this and as soon as he finishes his examination he'll explain as much as he can at this early stage.

There'll certainly be some tests that will have to be done, but in the meantime here are some of the questions you might like to ask:

- What does the doctor think it could be?
- What could be causing it?
- Is it something that can be cured?
- What will the treatment be?
- Is there anything that can be given now that will ease the pain/discomfort?
- What further tests will be needed and how long are they likely to take?
- Could it be something that's life threatening?

If your doctor feels that you might have a type of arthritis you may want to ask him if he thinks that, at this stage, it would be advisable for you to go along to a local support group. (See Chapter 11, page 99.)

The tests

Very rarely will your doctor be able to give you an immediate diagnosis of the problem and he will most probably ask for some tests to be done. He can either arrange for these himself, or refer you to a private rheumatologist or the rheumatology team at your local hospital. (See page 28.)

It's also rare for one single test to give an answer and it's likely that you'll need a series of them before a clear picture emerges. Let's take a look at some of these tests:

X-ray: An X-ray is a useful tool in detecting two of the most common forms of arthritis — osteoarthritis and rheumatoid arthritis — as it clearly shows any deterioration of the cartilage, the condition of the bone ends, decreased bone density and tissue swelling. If you've already had X-rays taken, even a long time ago, take them with you when you see your doctor.

Blood tests: Much useful information can be gathered by taking a close look at your blood. In many cases there'll need to be a number of different tests done before your doctor or rheumatologist can make a positive diagnosis of arthritis. The results of blood tests are looked at in relation to the other tests you've had and a diagnosis is made on the whole picture.

Most blood tests are referred to by the initials describing what they test for; for example, ANA (antinuclear antibodies), CBC (complete blood count), CRP (C-reactive protein), anti-CCP (anticyclic citrullinated peptide), ENA (extractable nuclear antigens), ESR (erythrocyte sedimentation rate), HLA-B27 human leucocyte antigen-B27 (the B refers to the B region in this gene. There are four regions: A, B, C and D).

MRI scan (magnetic resonance imaging): Taken by sophisticated machines that work by bringing together radio waves, magnetism and a computer, these images are particularly helpful in the early detection of osteoarthritis and rheumatoid arthritis as they are able to detect erosion in the joints that is too subtle to be picked up by X-ray.

CT scans (computerised tomography): Using a computer and X-ray technology, CT scans create a series of images that can be viewed as slices through the body.

Biopsy: By taking a sample of the joint lining or synovial membrane it is possible to tell why a joint is swollen or causing pain. Many types of arthritis can also be diagnosed by taking biopsies of muscle or skin.

Joint aspiration: Under a local anaesthetic, a small needle is inserted into the affected joint and fluid is withdrawn and sent to a laboratory for testing.

After all the tests have been completed and the results known, the chances are that you'll remain under the care of your doctor. However, if he considers that you need specialist care he may refer you to a rheumatologist, either privately or through your local hospital.

The rheumatologist

A rheumatologist is a doctor (physician, see below) who has specialised in the diagnosis and treatment of arthritis, disorders of the joints, muscles and soft tissues, and auto-immune diseases that do not affect any one specific organ system.

They will also see patients with generalised inflammatory or auto-immune diseases and pain arising from tendons, ligaments and other soft tissue structures around bones and joints.

What is a physician?

Historically, a doctor who has specialised in one of the medical disciplines is referred to as a physician and carries the title Doctor (Dr). Up until the twentieth century, surgeons were not trained at universities and therefore carried the term Mister (Mr).

Many patients like to keep a formal basis to the relationship by calling their rheumatologist 'Doctor', and being addressed in return as Mr or Mrs; others may prefer first names. Your rheumatologist is likely to be comfortable in either situation.

The hospital team

This is a dedicated specialist team within the hospital that takes a multi-disciplined approach to the care and wellbeing of people with arthritis.

On referring you to the hospital your doctor will have forwarded details of your arthritis and an appointment will be made for you depending on the urgency of your condition (the technical name for this decision-making process is *triage*).

Your first visit to the hospital will most probably be through the outpatients department where the staff will share your care with your doctor. But don't be surprised if they repeat some of the tests you've already had — it's part of their in-depth assessment process.

While you're being assessed you'll have access to the specialists who make up your treatment team. Depending on your condition and your need, here are some of the people you're likely to meet:

Rheumatologist: The leader of the team who'll be guiding your treatment.

Physiotherapist: This is the person who'll be working with you to reduce your pain, build your strength, increase your range of movement and help you put together your own exercise programme.

Occupational therapist: The person who will work with you and other members of the team to help draw up a long-term management plan and show you the special techniques and devices that will help you with your day-to-day activities. (See Chapter 11, page 95.)

Social worker: The person who can help you access those important community resources, such as local support groups, home help and, should you want it, counselling.

Dietitian: A dietitian will help you devise an eating plan made up of well-balanced nutrients best suited for your condition.

Pharmacist: Working with you and the rheumatologist, the pharmacist will ensure that you are being prescribed the most effective medication for your condition and will explain how you can maximise its efficiency and minimise any side effects.

Should your condition deteriorate while you're under the care of the hospital, you may need to be admitted to the inpatients ward for treatment and rehabilitation.

Arthritis educator: The arthritis educator is there to help you achieve a better quality of life through the following:

- Developing a positive approach to their disease and the challenges it creates
- Providing education and advice on prevention and management
- Facilitating access to relevant services and agencies
- Explaining what physical aids are available
- Developing a self-management strategy

Specialist rheumatology units

In some areas there are specialist rheumatology units where the rheumatologists work in conjunction with specialist rheumatology outpatients' nurses. The role of the nurse in such units is as follows:

- Educating patients as to the nature of the disease
- Helping them understand their own condition
- Monitoring blood and X-ray results
- Providing a holistic approach to their treatment
- Ensuring that patients understand the medication they're taking
- Showing patients how to manage and work on strategies for their pain relief
- Ensuring that patients realise the importance of keeping appointments, taking their medications and having their regular blood tests
- Helping the patient establish an exercise regime
- Making necessary referrals to other members of the team, such as physiotherapists and occupational therapists
- Discussing any family issues that may have arisen since the original diagnosis

If you live outside these areas you'll most likely be under the care of your doctor who'll put you in contact with one of the 33 arthritis educators who work under the umbrella of Arthritis New Zealand. (See Appendix 2, Useful contacts, page 115.)

The rheumatologist–doctor–nurse–patient relationship

If you have chronic inflammatory arthritis you may need to have regular follow-ups in the rheumatology outpatients department and, ideally, you will end up building a good working relationship with your rheumatologist and the rheumatology nurse. Such a relationship may last many years and it's hoped that during that time a strong degree of mutual trust and respect will have been built between you all.

At the beginning, you may feel that you have no control and that all decisions have been taken out of your hands. This may of course be true, for until you understand your condition and your body's reaction to the medication you're taking, you must remember that what is being suggested is what is considered best for you. As time goes by and you understand your condition — perhaps even better than the medical team — your input will be of great value and significance in deciding how your treatment should continue.

Issues that are likely to be ongoing between you, your rheumatologist and the all-important nurse are:

Medications: This includes a review of the medication you're taking and whether or not it is suppressing your immune system and gaining control of the disease. (See Appendix 4, page 126.)

Blood tests: The results of your blood tests will be reviewed at each appointment to see how well the medication is supressing the inflammatory process and to monitor possible side effects in the liver and blood cells.

Symptoms that may be present: Sometimes painful and swollen joints (particularly knees) may need draining if there's fluid present. Once the fluid is drained an injection of a steroid is given into the joint and this generally settles down the inflammation so that the joint can return to normal within a few days.

Any new problems that have developed: If you are experiencing a restricted range of movement with some joints, you may need to be referred to a physiotherapist to help you maintain function and flexibility in your joints.

Pain levels: Patients with arthritis are usually very stoic, putting up with a great deal of pain while saying very little about it. However, honesty is more important than bravery and it's only by knowing your real pain levels that your medical team can make the alterations to your medication that will give you the best possible quality of life.

Keeping a journal

Keeping a record of how you've been feeling can be a great help to your doctors in monitoring the progress of your arthritis. All you need is a small notebook in which to keep a record of your symptoms, changes in medication and any other information relevant to your condition.

Chapter 3

Developing your management plan

The doctors have asked all their questions, you've been poked, prodded and examined from head to toe, the tests have been done and you've now been diagnosed as having a form of arthritis. Where to from here?

Our experience has shown that most people with arthritis find it much easier to cope with their day-to-day activities if they develop and put in place a structured management strategy. Yes, there will be limitations to your activities, but with careful planning and management these can be minimised. And yes, there may be certain sports or hobbies you'll no longer be able to enjoy, but as one door shuts, so often another opens and you might well surprise yourself with what you find in your new world. So many people who have to cope with arthritis tell us how much they're enjoying new pastimes and interests that they would never have thought of or considered.

But, before we start looking at the elements that make up a structured management plan, let's take a close look at what the central part of any plan will be — the relief of pain.

As it's not easy to be happy or contented if you're hurting, the first thing we have to look at is to do something about your pain — and to satisfactorily do that we must begin by first understanding what pain is and what's causing it.

What is pain?

Put very simply, pain is the message that's being sent through your nerve pathways to your brain to tell you that some part of your body has been hurt and to ask you to please do something about it. There are two very different pain messages:

Acute pain: This is a message of warning; for example, if you fall and twist your ankle, a message will immediately be sent off to your brain and you'll feel pain and do something about it. Acute pain comes on quickly, builds up to a peak and then slowly tapers off. Its purpose is to get you to do something about it, and when you do, the pain subsides.

Chronic pain: This is the pain that emanates from a part of the inner body when it's been damaged, not by a sudden event, but rather by an internal illness or disease such as arthritis. It doesn't come on quickly, but is there all the time trying to tell the brain that something is wrong. Unlike the twisted ankle, the damage isn't temporary and so the message is sent over and over and over again — like an insistent telephone that isn't being answered, it's this pain that arthritis sufferers experience.

Managing chronic pain

The key to managing chronic pain is to find ways to block or slow down the pain messages as they make their way to the brain. Medication is of course one way (we discuss this in Appendix 4, page 126) but there are many other things that can be done.

The gate theory of pain

In the mid 1960s two scientists developed what we call the 'gate theory of pain' — they put forward the idea that there were 'gates' along our nerve pathways which could, depending on certain conditions, open or close, thereby either allowing pain messages to get through, or delaying them.

What is particularly interesting about this theory is that it's our minds and emotions that have this control over the movements of the gates. If we feel stressed, angry or depressed the gates tend to open and let the pain messages through. However, the less stressed, angry or depressed we are, the more the gates tend to close, letting less of the pain message through.

So what can you do to try and keep those mysterious gates as near to closed as possible? Unfortunately, there's no one catch-all answer, as not everyone responds to everything in the same way. To a certain extent, it's a matter of finding what's right for you. (See Chapter 11, page 88.)

The pain cycle

Many people when first diagnosed with arthritis quite naturally feel frustrated and angry. This can lead to them feeling stressed, which in turn — anger plus stress — can only too often lead to depression.

Unfortunately, those three emotions — anger, stress and depression — we now know are the very emotions that adversely influence the 'pain gates' and have a strong bearing on how we feel pain. Sadly, they make it worse!

With increased pain, frustration and anger increase, we become more stressed, more depressed . . . and so more pain, more stress, more anger, yet again more pain . . . and so the cycle starts. Once the cycle starts it's difficult to break.

!! The earlier you can break this cycle, or better still not allow it to develop, the easier your life will be.

Assessing your options

Once your condition has been diagnosed you'll sit with your rheumatologist and he'll go over the various treatment options that need to be considered. (If your symptoms are mild and you can put up with them and they don't interfere with your daily living, you may not need to have treatment.)

Though every form of arthritis is different and has its own treatment depending on the individual, each responds to a number of universal courses of action. Let's have a look at these.

Medication

The chances are that up until now you've been on a course of pain relief and anti-inflammatory medication. Now that the cause of the problem is known, your medication can be modified, to not only give pain relief but also to act upon the problem itself. (We'll take a close look at the various medications in Appendix 4, page 126.)

Change of lifestyle

To successfully manage your arthritis you may have to make some changes in your lifestyle. While your arthritis may limit some of your past activities, with the right management programme there is still much you can do to ensure that you have a rewarding and fulfilled life. The areas of change that you'll have to look at are:

Physical therapy: You'll be surprised just how much a little bit of exercise each day can help — discuss with your team the exercises that best suit your condition and together draw up a suitable programme. (In Chapter 9, page 69, we'll look at the various options, from the benefits of walking to the delights of aqua-jogging.)

Diet: By simply changing to a healthy, balanced diet that consists of a balance of the foods your body needs — carbohydrates, proteins, minerals and vitamins — you'll find it much easier to maintain a positive attitude. (We'll look at this in Chapter 10, page 77.)

Stress management: Stress in itself is neither harmful nor dangerous — what causes us problems is the way we react to it. (In Chapter 11, page 89 we'll take a look at stress, discuss what causes it, and offer some suggestions that will help you manage it.)

The power of the mind: Every day at the hospital clinic we see patients who, by taking a positive attitude, are managing to cope with their condition and are living satisfying lives — we cannot stress strongly enough just how important it is that you look at and concentrate on the things you *can* do rather than those you *can't*. (See Chapter 12, page 101.)

Splints and supports

Splints: For temporary relief of joint pain you can use a splint. Normally made of plastic and rubber, they can be fitted to an affected joint to allow it to rest. The benefits of a splint are:

- Easing of pain
- Keeping inflammation under control
- Helping to keep the joint in position, preventing deformities

Supports: Also available for temporary relief of pain, these are strong elastic wraps that fit over and around wrists, ankles, knees, etc.

Splints and supports are available through medical supply shops. They can also be tailor-made to fit — talk to your occupational therapist about the best option for your condition.

Surgery

As surgery always carries a certain risk it will only be considered after all other avenues — medication, diet, physiotherapy, and pain management strategies — have been thoroughly explored. Your rheumatologist will then discuss the situation with you, and the possibility of referring you to an *orthopaedic surgeon*. (See also Chapter 4, page 39.)

Complementary therapies

These include any treatment undertaken in conjunction with your conventional medical care that you find eases your pain or discomfort and doesn't harm other parts of your body.

Complementary therapies take many forms and range from acupuncture, through homeopathy to yoga. Some, such as meditation, may not in themselves ease your pain, but will work wonders helping you relax, which in turn is what will have an influence on your pain. Equally, t'ai chi, with its slow rhythmic movements, will lower your stress levels while at the same time giving you improved arm and leg function and bending ability.

!! *Complementary therapies are not to be confused with alternative therapies which are often offered in place of traditional medical treatment.*

Some of the more common alternative therapies are:

Acupressure: Similar to acupuncture but fingers and hands are used instead of needles. Acupressure is sometimes called *shiatsu.*

Acupuncture: A major part of Chinese medicine, acupuncture has been around for thousands of years treating disease through balancing the body's energy flow. The Chinese theory is that we each have 12 lines of energy (*meridians*) running through our bodies and it's when these 'channels' become blocked, restricting the flow of energy, that we experience pain and disease.

By stimulating some of the *acupuncture points* along the meridians, the acupuncturist will unblock the obstruction and re-establish the flow of energy. This stimulation can be done in the following manner using very fine, hair-thin needles: a small amount of herb (*mugwort*) is burned over the acupuncture point before inserting the needles, then a low current is put through the needles after insertion.

Acupuncture also stimulates the immune and circulatory systems releasing your own natural painkillers — endorphins.

Alexander technique: Based on the premise that many of our ills and problems stem from incorrect posture, this technique teaches you to stand and move in ways that put minimum stress on your body.

Aromatherapy: This ancient art uses fragrant substances called *essential oils* to treat the ills of the mind and body. The oils are put into boiling water and the fumes inhaled. Essential oils you might try are *camomile, eucalyptus* and *ginger*.

Chiropractic: A system of treating disorders by manipulating the spine and other parts of the body.

Hydrotherapy: If you've ever lain back in a tub full of hot water you'll know the benefits of hydrotherapy. In certain circumstances, cold water or ice can be equally beneficial.

Massage: Massage is the act of manipulating the body by kneading, pressing or stroking affected areas. The benefits of massage are a temporary feeling of wellbeing and reduced pain resulting from the increased level of endorphins.

Medicinal herbs: Before the development of doctors and pharmacists, our early ancestors learned that certain plants stimulated their bodies to a sense of wellbeing. Though we've come a long way since then in our medical understanding, many people still find comfort in the use of herbs.

Meditation: Expanding self-awareness by deep concentrated thought, practitioners use the experience to strengthen positive thinking and eliminate the negative.

Pilates: The Pilates teacher uses a thorough understanding of the anatomy of the human body to create a comprehensive exercise programme for each individual, with the aim of restoring a greater sense of 'balance'. It is this holistic approach that sets Pilates apart from many other forms of exercise.

T'ai chi ch'uan: Usually known by its shortened name, t'ai chi, meaning wellness, this is a series of slow-moving, dance-like movements, which encourage body awareness, balance and the presence of self. It was developed by Taoist monks who combined movement with special breathing techniques as a way of integrating body, mind and spirit.

Perhaps t'ai chi is the reason why so many Chinese live to a ripe old age.

Yoga: The word 'yoga' comes from the Sanskrit for 'yoke' or 'union'. Its underlying philosophy is to bring our mind, body and spirit into a state of balance and harmony. It is made up of a series of related exercises and postures, called *asanas*. The benefits to be enjoyed from yoga are improved flexibility, increased energy, improved circulation and reduced stress.

!! *You are strongly advised to discuss any plans to undertake complementary therapies with your doctor or rheumatologist.*

Chapter 4

Surgery

Just because an operation can be done doesn't mean it should be done and sometimes conservative treatments are more appropriate. Therefore, only a small percentage of patients with arthritis will end up having orthopaedic surgery.

Whether you should have an operation or not will depend on a number of factors including: the impact of the arthritis on your life; the likely success of the operation; your age (you can be too young as well as too old); your general health; and your response to less-invasive treatments.

While surgery has the potential to transform peoples' lives for the better, there are also certain risks. If the element of risk concerns you, why not go along for an assessment and discussion with the surgeon. Remember, nobody can force you to have an operation you don't want, and the more you know, the better you'll be able to make a decision that's right for you. So don't be afraid to ask questions and if you'd feel more comfortable, take someone along with you. Some questions you might ask are:

- What surgery is being recommended?
- Can you please describe the procedure?
- Are there potential complications?
- What is the success rate?
- How will I be better off?
- How long will I be in hospital?
- How long will I be off work?

Types of surgery

Surgery has an important role to play in the lives of many patient who have arthritis, though not before a full conservative treatmen programme has been trialled, which would have included advice or arthritis, getting your weight down, medication, physiotherapy and provision of helpful aids. Many people think of joint arthroplasty (tota joint replacements) as the ultimate surgical procedure but there are many other operations.

Arthroscopy: This involves the insertion of a telescope into a join allowing it to be examined, but more importantly, the washing out o some inflammatory fluids and trimming of excess or degenerate tissue This may include meniscus (in the knee), and articular cartilage or sca tissue in other joints.

Arthrotomy: Literally, this means 'opening a joint with a surgica incision'. Again, this can lead to trimming of any damaged or exces tissue or, sometimes, even the removal of a damaged joint.

Synovectomy: The removal of the inflammatory lining of joint and tendon sheaths allows better function (movement) and loss of the associated pain.

Osteotomy: The surgical division of a bone (usually at a poin adjacent to a joint) corrects any abnormal angulation of the associated bones. This can alter the pressure loading through a joint, especially around the knee but also it sometimes has a healing effect on the associated joint. The bone will then heal the same way as a fracture o break. (Often the joint is held in position with screws and plates or a plaster cast for a time to allow healing to occur.)

Arthrodesis: This involves surgical stiffening of a joint. Usually, a joint is set in a physiologically correct anatomical position and has the advantage of removing pain from the affected joint. The disadvantage i that the joint doesn't move and, theoretically, can put extra stresses or adjacent mobile joints. Arthrodesis is a useful operation in some spina conditions, the fingers, the wrists, the ankles, feet and toes.

Excision arthroplasty: This involves washing out the damage joint, especially in the feet and toes.

Replacement arthroplasty: Many joints can now be replaced including shoulders, elbows, wrists, fingers, spine, hips, knees and ankles.

When is surgery indicated?

Surgery is usually considered after all other medical treatments have been exhausted. However, occasionally it may be used earlier; for example, in the case of tendon rupture and inflammatory arthritis. There are a number of factors that might indicate that surgery is a realistic option for you:

Pain: This is the main indication. Patients with arthritic joints are aware of sharp, catching pain due to the mechanical stress or rubbing of the joint but they may also often experience a dull, deep pain especially at night. Unrelieved night pain is one of the main indications for joint replacement.

Stiffness: Scarring and fibrosis around an arthritic joint can limit movement. Poor muscle tone and fears of joint pain will also interfere with active use of the joint.

Instability: When the joint surface is destroyed the ligaments can become lax and the joint can become unstable, particularly the knee. This can also occur because loose pieces of bone, called 'loose bodies', float around joints.

Deformity: When a joint suffers significant damage, it may become asymmetrical leading to deformity of the joint. Muscle spasm, secondary to pain, can also cause joint deformity.

Loss of function: Activities of daily living may become difficult with an arthritic joint. Surgery can often help.

Medical aspects of orthopaedic surgery

The decision on whether surgery is the best treatment for your arthritis will depend on a number of factors, not the least of which is your general health. If you suffer from a serious medical condition, especially one affecting the heart and lungs, the risks of surgery may outweigh the benefits. An anaesthetist will generally make this decision, but you may need to be assessed by another specialist.

Some medications will need to be withheld around the time of surgery, particularly drugs that thin the blood, such as aspirin and warfarin; your anaesthetist and surgeon will advise you on this and some surgeons may prefer their patients to withhold other arthritis medications such as methotrexate. This will not usually result in a serious flare of arthritis if the time gap for treatment is no greater than three weeks, but you may be advised to discuss this with your rheumatologist if your surgeon is recommending a longer period than this.

Total joint replacement

Hundreds of thousands of patients around the world each year benefit from joint replacement (arthroplasty). The first successful total joint replacements were developed 50 years ago and there have been many changes since, some of which, unfortunately, have proved unsatisfactory.

Most replacements have bearing surfaces roughly similar to the original joint and at least one part is made of metal — either stainless steel or an alloy. Titanium has been largely superseded because it has poor wear characteristics, although it is excellent for bone in-growth. Many artificial joints also have a plastic component (high-density polyethylene) or ceramic surfaces. All have their advantages and disadvantages.

There are many variations, especially in hip and knee replacements. The aim is to get as little friction as possible between the joint surfaces, but no artificial bearing can compare with the articular cartilage in a normal joint, which offers very low friction (less than a skate sliding on ice).

Plastic bearing-surfaces have now been used for many years but they do wear and the small particles that are released can cause loosening of the components in the bone. Metal-on-metal prostheses have much better wear characteristics, but it is a theoretical worry that metal ions that are released into the body may be harmful long term. Ceramics have very low friction but there is a very small possibility of fracture releasing very abrasive particles into the joint.

For many years all components were cemented into the bone. Uncemented in-growth components are now available with a rough surface allowing the bone to grow into the prosthesis.

Recently, minimally invasive surgery (MIS), which involves replacement of the bearing surfaces only, has become fashionable. This is still experimental and there are many complications associated with this procedure though the scar is small and rehabilitation is said to be quicker. Surface replacement aims to protect some of the normal bony architecture, but the jury is still out regarding its long-term effectiveness.

When your medical advisor recommends an operation you'll have appointments with a pre-operative nurse, a physiotherapist, an occupational therapist and an anaesthetist.

A general medical check is important, particularly concerning your skin condition and any underlying source of infection; for example, in your urinary system.

You may have a spinal or general anaesthetic depending on the preference of the operating team.

Post-operatively, it is important that you listen to the instructions you'll be given. Many people listen to what their friends have told them but they may be discussing a different operation with a different surgical procedure.

Complications of total joint replacement

Most patients are middle aged or older so general health becomes important and some medications may need to be modified. However, there are a number of other specific concerns to be considered.

Venous thrombosis: Operations on the lower limbs are liable to affect the circulation in the venous system, which is made up of the vessels that carry blood back to the heart after it's been through the arteries. Circulation can become sluggish and a clot may form causing obstruction and swelling in the leg. If a piece of such a clot breaks free it can travel to the chest and cause a pulmonary embolism. This risk can be lessened by being fit pre-operatively, elevating your lower limbs post-operatively, starting exercise soon after and, possibly, by using blood-thinning medication (anticoagulants).

Dislocation: In the first few weeks following surgery stability of the components (particularly in a hip replacement) depend on the surrounding muscles. Any sudden movement, particularly in an awkward position, can cause the ball to come out of the socket. It is important that you listen to instructions regarding methods for reducing this risk. In the majority of dislocation cases, the ball can be put back in the socket and the post-operative rehabilitation will progress satisfactorily.

Leg-length discrepancy: However much care is taken by the surgeon it is sometimes difficult to get exact leg-length equality post-operatively, because the muscles and other tissues must be balanced around the replacement.

Infection: The skin is always contaminated and there is a slight risk of organisms being introduced at the time of surgery in spite of prophylactic antibiotics and other precautions. This is often caused by a normally non-virulent organism, but, because of the tissue damage and the foreign material, the body can't always control this infection. It may not be evident for several months after surgery.

Infection can also occur at a later stage, secondary to other infections in the body that travel in the blood and settle in the joint replacement. It is therefore important to take long-term care of any ulcers or infections, particularly in the legs. Acute infections elsewhere in the body; for example, the gall bladder, the urinary tract, or the lung, should also be treated aggressively to prevent them settling in the joint replacement.

Prosthesis wear: The replacement is like any other machine and, if you live long enough, will eventually wear out. Small wear particles travel away from the joints and pass between the surrounding bone and the prosthesis, stimulating a secretion of enzymes that cause loosening. Plastic components can wear out and break-up, so requiring a new replacement joint. You should treat your prosthesis carefully and you'll be given advice at the time of surgery of the level of activity which you should expect. Revision of most prostheses is possible, but it is a more difficult operation with more complications and less chance of success.

Peri-prosthetic fracture: The products of loosening can weaken the bone around a prosthesis. The metal components have different stress characteristics from the bone and occasionally the bone can fracture around a prosthesis. Sometimes this is a stress fracture but can also occur as a result of trauma.

In spite of these complications the vast majority of joint replacements are successful. It's very easy to forget that you've been given a replacement but you should make sure that you have regular post-operative checks at intervals suggested by your surgeon.

Will I set off security systems?

Security screening is not an X-ray as many people think, but a beam that is deflected by metal. Most prostheses don't register as they're buried within the tissues, though occasionally the sensitivity of the detector is altered and you may be stopped. If you have a joint replacement you should be given a card, which you should always carry with you and show if necessary.

Post-operative care

Following public hospital surgery

Prior to discharge from the ward, nursing staff or the ward social worker will sit with you and develop a discharge plan. This will include referrals to any support services you may require on either a short- or long-term basis. This includes rehabilitation therapies such as:

- Home help
- Assistance with personal cares
- Physiotherapy
- Special equipment

It is important that this is organised before your discharge, so if you're unsure whether it's been organised, ask the nursing staff and, if necessary, they'll arrange it for you. If the discharge plan isn't developed or if, when you get home, you find you need additional assistance you'll need to visit your GP for a referral to the Community Rehabilitation Team, which consists of the following specialists:

- Occupational therapists
- Social workers
- Physiotherapists
- Other relevant health professionals

Following private hospital surgery

If you have your operation in a private hospital you will need to make the arrangements for your post-operative care before you go into hospital. If, for any reason, this is not possible, the nurse or support staff on the ward will either make referrals to the appropriate support services or directly to your own GP.

!! Whether you're in a public or private hospital it's very important that you have the required support services set up prior to leaving the hospital. If you're not sure this has been done ask the nursing staff.

Part two

Types of arthritis

True or false?

Osteoporosis is a form of arthritis.
False
Although osteoporosis affects the bones it is not a form of arthritis.

Your doctor can tell if you have arthritis through
blood tests and X-rays.
True
However, this is not true for all types of arthritis.

Arthritis can get worse if not treated.
True
That's why it's so important to diagnose it as early as possible.

Chapter 5

Osteoarthritis

This chapter deals exclusively with the condition of osteoarthritis and should be read in conjunction with the information in the body of the book.

Also known as degenerative arthritis or degenerative joint disease, osteoarthritis (OA) is the most common form of arthritis affecting between 10 and 20 per cent of people over the age of 65. It's the only form of arthritis that we bring upon ourselves, through no other reason than the fact that we use, and put pressure on, our joints. (See Chapter 1, page 17.) The areas most commonly affected are the neck, lower back, hips, knees, hands, ankles and toes.

In OA, the cartilage that sits between the bones in our joints becomes roughened and wears down. In advanced cases the cartilage can wear

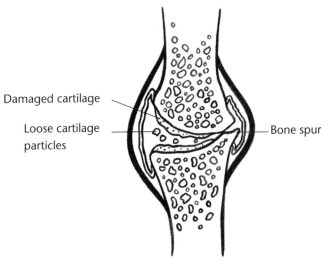

A joint damaged due to osteoarthritis.

down completely so that bone rubs on bone causing spurs called *osteophytes* to form around the ends of the joint. These can often be seen and felt as bony lumps around the damaged area.

The symptoms of osteoarthritis

The primary indicators of OA are:

- **Joint pain** — the initial feeling is an ache that becomes stronger as the joints are used — at first it will generally lessen with rest though over time it can become quite steady
- **Stiffness** — often coupled with restricted movement
- **Swelling** — mostly seen in the fingers and knees

Having any of the above symptoms doesn't necessarily mean you have OA, but it should be enough of an indication for you to have a talk with your doctor.

What causes osteoarthritis?

There are two categories of osteoarthritis (OA):

Primary arthritis: This is when we don't know what triggered the cartilage to corrode. Scientists believe, but have yet to prove, that enzymes damage the fibres that hold the cartilage together causing it to become weak and lose its structure.

Secondary arthritis: This is when we know what the likely trigger was — most commonly one of the following:

- **Trauma (injury)** — includes any injury to one of your joints, most likely through sports' activity or a car accident. (You don't have to be carried off the field with a joint injury, the damage can accumulate with pressure that is repetitive over a number of years.)
- **Being overweight** — carrying excess weight is an invitation to OA to visit your weight-bearing joints; e.g. hips, knees and ankles
- **Repetitive motion** — when certain joints are put to repeated use, you're likely to court OA, e.g. footballers' knees

- **Bone damage** — a car accident that results in bone damage commonly leads to OA

Who is at risk?

Not everyone is destined to get arthritis and there are many octogenarians who can whisk around as if they were young teenagers. But we're not all that fortunate and our chances of developing OA are increased if we fall into one or more of the following categories:

Age: The dangerous years seem to be between 45 and 55. It isn't age itself that causes the problem, but rather the decades of use (and abuse) that you have put your joints through.

Weight: Carrying around extra kilos puts too much stress on your joints and eventually the cartilage will be damaged.

Gender: Women are much more likely to develop OA than men, particularly among the older age group.

Repeated use: Many jobs require repeated use of certain joints and after a number of years the cartilage in those joints can become excessively worn, resulting in the development of arthritis.

Genes: Not everyone whose mother or father had arthritis will develop the disease. However, if there is arthritis in your family tree, there'll be a predisposition for you to also develop it.

Injury: If one of your joints is injured in your youth; for example, through playing sport or a minor accident, there is the possibility that you'll develop OA in later life.

Treatment

Quite often you may find that the only treatment you'll need when your joints are painful is simply to rest. Gentle exercises to strengthen the muscles around your joints, especially the knee, should help keep the pain at bay. (See page 55 and Chapter 9, page 69.)

If you feel that resting isn't easing your pain you can try the following medications:

- Take some paracetamol and, if that isn't sufficient, you can add one of the non-steroidal anti-inflammatory drugs. (See Appendix 4, page 128.)
- The dietary supplements glucosamine and chondroitin

have been shown to reduce pain, although the effect may depend on the brand. *Capsaicin cream* appears to reduce pain when applied directly to the affected joint

- An injection of the steroid *cortisone* into the affected joint will often give you prolonged relief
- If you have OA in the knee, more prolonged relief may be achieved with an injection of *Synvisc®*

If these measures don't relieve your pain and keep you mobile, have a talk with your doctor about the possibility of surgery. (See Chapter 4, page 39.)

There is a comprehensive list of medications in Appendix 4, page 126.

!! Drugs whose names start with a lowercase letter are generic; brand names always start with a capital letter.

Chapter 6

Rheumatoid arthritis

This chapter deals exclusively with the condition of rheumatoid arthritis and should be read in conjunction with the information in the body of the book.

Rheumatoid arthritis (RA) is the most common form of inflammatory arthritis and it's estimated that it affects approximately two to three per cent of New Zealanders.

The symptoms of rheumatoid arthritis

Although the symptoms of RA are similar to those of osteoarthritis (see Chapter 5, page 50), the diseases are very different. In the early stages RA symptoms may be mistaken for those of osteoarthritis — joint pain, stiffness and swelling — but soon differences become apparent. For example, joints are affected in a symmetrical manner — both hands, both knees, both elbows, etc.

As RA is a systemic disease, though predominantly in one of the joints, it can also trigger problems in other parts of the body, such as eyes, heart and lungs. The following symptoms may develop:

- *Rheumatoid nodules*, small lumps under the skin may appear, particularly, but not exclusively, in elbows and feet
- Dryness of the eyes and mouth
- A general feeling of tiredness and nausea

If the disease isn't controlled and is allowed to progress it may result in permanent deformity and loss of function.

What causes rheumatoid arthritis?

RA results when a normally efficient immune system, for reasons we don't yet fully understand, runs amok and attacks the *synovial membrane* in your joints.

While there are many theories as to why our immune system should make such an assault on the body it's protecting, we don't yet have a simple explanation.

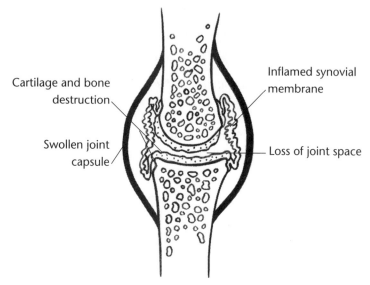

Cartilage and bone destruction

Inflamed synovial membrane

Swollen joint capsule

Loss of joint space

A joint damaged due to rheumatoid arthritis.

Who is at risk?

The unfortunate answer for half the population is that the disease shows no favouritism to age, colour, creed or race, with one exception. For reasons not well understood, women are more than twice as likely as men to get the disease.

The tests for rheumatoid arthritis

As early symptoms don't always show themselves at the same time, RA can be extremely difficult to diagnose and your doctor may have to arrive at a diagnosis by way of eliminating other possible causes. Many significant symptoms may not be apparent for months and sometimes years, so the diagnostic process could take quite some time. (See Chapter 2, page 23.)

Specific tests for the presence of RA are as follows:

Blood tests: *Red blood cell count* (RBC), checking for anaemia; *Rheumatic factor test* (RF) and *anti-CCP antibodies* — these are not necessarily conclusive as they can also show positive in other diseases and in healthy people; *Erythrocyte sedimentation rate (ESR)*, testing for the presence of inflammation.

X-ray: The affected joints are X-rayed for damage to bone and/or cartilage.

Joint fluid sample: A sample of joint fluid is taken to test for inflammation.

Treatment

The principal treatment for RA is medication which is aimed at reducing pain and controlling inflammation. The main types of drugs used are listed below.

NSAIDs (non-steroidal anti-inflammatory drugs): These reduce swelling and relieve pain. Two common examples are *aspirin* and *ibuprofen*.

DMARDs (disease modifying anti-rheumatic drugs): These will improve symptoms in the short term and reduce the risk of damage in the longer term. The choice of DMARD depends on individual circumstances, but is usually between *sulphasalazine* (Salazopyrine) and *methotrexate*. If either of these is ineffective by itself, the two can be combined. Other options include *leflunomide* (Arava), and a milder agent *hydroxychloroquine* (Plaquenil) may be added to the treatment.

The next line of defence is the gold injections (Myocrisin), *azathioprine* or *cyclosporine* (Neoral).

Biologic response modifiers: This new class of drug is used for severe cases that have failed to respond to other treatments. Examples include: *etanercept* (Enbrel*), *infliximab* (Remicade*) and *adalimumab* (Humira).

Corticosteroids (steroids): As DMARDs take two to three months to be effective, corticosteroids are often used in limited courses early on in order to bring the disease under control. The most common is *prednisone.*

Even with the best possible medical treatment, over time the joints may become damaged. The option then is surgery which will either correct any deformity or replace worn and damaged joints. (See Chapter 4, page 39.)

Chapter 7

Gout

This chapter deals exclusively with the condition of gout and should be read in conjunction with the information in the body of the book.

The common picture of gout is of a portly gentleman, glass in hand, sitting in his club, one foot bandaged like a rugby ball and resting on a stately cushion. The reality is somewhat different. Although it is more common in men, gout can affect anyone irrespective of gender, class or standing.

The symptoms of gout

One of the distinctive features of gout is that it can suddenly appear with no warning and cause you agonising pain, more often than not starting in the joint at the base of your big toe.

If not showing itself in the big toe, it can appear in any other joint, although the spine, shoulder and hips are rarely affected.

What causes gout?

Gout is a disease in which inflammation and damage to bones and joints is caused by the deposit of needle-shaped crystals of *uric acid* in the soft tissues of the affected joint.

When the uric acid in the blood exceeds a certain level, crystals form, and the white blood cells, attempting to remove these crystals, release inflammatory products that cause the typical symptoms of swelling, redness, heat and pain.

In the early stages, the symptoms can come on rapidly with great intensity, though they will usually settle between bouts. In the later stages, the symptoms may be milder but with little relief between attacks. Deposits of uric acid crystals may form into small lump-like clusters called *tophi* (the plural of *tophus*) in the tissues.

Who is at risk?

As most of the uric acid our body produces is derived from what we eat, so an excessive intake of *purines* (see page 58) is often an important causative factor and will put you at risk.

Other risk factors include:

- Excessive alcohol intake (especially beer, which is worse for gout than port or red wine)
- Ethnicity (Maori and Pacific people are more at risk)
- Family history
- High blood pressure
- Other diseases, including kidney disease, heart disease and diabetes

There is a particular type of gout that occurs in elderly patients, usually female, who are taking diuretic medication for heart failure and high blood pressure. The uric acid level in their blood can be very high and there may be a rapid deposit of tophi, especially in the fingers and often around osteoarthritic joints.

The tests for gout

Quite often the symptoms of gout are so clear that the diagnosis is obvious. Even so, your doctor will want to be sure and will instigate the following tests:

- Examination of fluid taken from the affected joint
- A blood test to check the levels of uric acid and find out if there are any lumps of uric acid crystals
- An X-ray of the joint

Treatment

In its early stages gout can be treated by avoiding the foods and drinks that trigger attacks, and by taking NSAIDs, *colchicine* and *corticosteroids* to relieve inflammation.

If the frequency of attacks increases, or if there's concern that tophi may be forming, *allopurinol* will often be prescribed to lower the level of uric acid in the blood.

!! Allopurinol *should not be started during an acute attack, and should be introduced gradually, making sure that it isn't going to cause an acute attack.*

How you can help

Luckily there's quite a lot that you can do to help heal your gout and prevent it from recurring:

- Cut back on the foods that contain *purines* (see below)
- Cut out alcohol, especially beer
- Keep your blood pressure down
- Exercise regularly
- Lose weight

Purines and food

Purines are one of the two types of building blocks of DNA — purines and pyrimidines. They are found in every living cell, including in our bodies and food.

Foods that are rich in *purines* and which you should avoid if you have gout are:

- Red meat, fatty meat, wild game
- Shellfish and oily fish — sardines, mackerel, herring, anchovies
- Offal — liver, kidneys, brains
- Marmite and Vegemite

Chapter 8

Other forms of arthritis

This chapter should be read in conjunction with the information in the body of the book.

Psoriatic arthritis (PsA)

Psoriatic arthritis is an inflammatory arthritis that affects about seven per cent of people who have the skin condition *psoriasis*.

Symptoms

In PsA, the joints of the fingers and toes may become inflamed and swollen (*dactylitis*) and in severe cases they may become deformed. It's also possible that other joints may be involved such as the spine and hips. When a lot of small and large joints are affected, and there is no spinal involvement, PsA can be difficult to distinguish from rheumatoid arthritis, though rheumatoid factor (an antibody found in the blood of 70 per cent of patients with rheumatoid arthritis) is not usually found in people with PsA.

Treatment

The treatment of PsA is very similar to that for rheumatoid arthritis. Analgesics and NSAIDs are the first line of treatment. If these measures are ineffective or if there is concern that joint damage may develop then DMARDs such as *methotrexate, sulphasalazine* and *leflunomide* are used.

If there is spinal involvement, permanent loss of movement may be prevented with exercise and NSAIDs. Joint injections may be useful, especially if there are only one or two affected joints.

Spondyloarthropathy (SpA)

This refers to a family of inflammatory arthritic conditions. People with these conditions often have a predisposing gene called HLA-B27. The list includes:

Ankylosing spondylitis (AS)

AS is most likely to affect men between the ages of 20 and 40 and attacks the cartilage, ligaments and tendons of the spine. The majority of patients have the gene HLA-B27, which also predisposes them to *iritis* (an inflammatory eye disease).

Symptoms

AS appears gradually as stiffness and pain in the lower back; it can be more noticeable at night and then ease as you become mobile. Other indications are loss of appetite, tiredness, fever and eye problems.

Treatment

The main aim of treatment is to ease the pain and prevent damage occurring to the spine — you're likely to be prescribed NSAIDs. Though damage can't be undone, physical exercise can help in preventing further harm.

Reactive arthritis

Generally affecting men between the ages of 20 and 50, reactive arthritis is triggered by bacterial infection of the stomach and urinary tract and tends to involve the large joints of the legs. It can also stem from a venereal infection.

Symptoms

These can fall into one or more of three groups:

> **Group 1:** Symptoms of arthritis — primarily pain and inflammation in the feet, ankles and knees, though it can also affect fingers, wrists and other joints
>
> **Group 2:** Symptoms of conjunctivitis — red, itchy and watery eyes
>
> **Group 3:** Inflammation of the *urethra*

Other symptoms may include rashes on hands or feet, and sores in the mouth or on genitalia. Many patients recover within 12 months although some symptoms of arthritis may persist.

Treatment

Antibiotics are given for the infection and NSAIDs for the inflammation and pain and, depending on your condition, your doctor may also prescribe stronger drugs, exercise and possibly eye drops for the conjunctivitis.

Enteropathic arthritis

This arthritis affects people who suffer from *Crohn's disease* and *ulcerative colitis* (an inflammatory condition of the bowel).

Symptoms

The symptoms are similar to those of reactive arthritis and psoriatic arthritis.

Treatment

The treatment is similar to reactive and psoriatic arthritis, but sometimes it's helpful to choose a DMARD that helps treat both the joint and the bowel diseases.

> ### Managing inflammatory spinal disease
>
> The general principle for managing inflammatory spinal disease is to reduce stiffness and pain with an NSAID and to prevent permanent loss of spinal movement with specific stretching exercises. Inflammation of the peripheral joints is treated with steroid injections and DMARDs as described for RA and PsA.

Auto-immune connective tissue diseases

In these diseases the immune system reacts against a variety of different tissues, often including those of the joints, skin, blood cells, kidneys, lungs and muscles. Patients with these diseases frequently have antibodies that attack body tissue. There is quite a lot of overlap in the features and symptoms of these diseases.

Systemic lupus erythematosis

Commonly called lupus or SLE, this disease can involve several organ systems and is most common in women during their childbearing years.

Symptoms

The characteristic features are:

- A rash in sun-exposed areas, especially across the cheeks (known as 'butterfly rash')
- The non-erosive arthritis symptoms of rheumatoid arthritis
- Symptoms of *Sjögren's syndrome* (see below) — dry eyes and mouth
- Symptoms of *Raynaud's phenomenon* (see page 63) — blanching then reddening of the fingers in the cold, low blood-cell count and inflammatory disease of the lungs, kidney and brain

Not all of these features need be present at the same time, and there is great variation in the severity of disease between individual cases.

Treatment

There are as many treatments as there are variations of the disease.

Discoid lupus erythematosus

This is a mild form of lupus that shows itself as a rash, typically appearing around the face, scalp and ears but may also be seen on the shoulders and the back of the arms.

Sjögren's syndrome

Primarily a disease of the salivary and tear glands, Sjögren's syndrome can occur on its own or together with one of the other auto-immune diseases, in particular RA and lupus.

Symptoms

Dryness of the eyes and mouth is the main symptom, but there may also be joint problems and sometimes a disease of the lungs, kidneys, brain and blood vessels (*vasculitis*). There is also the possibility of dental decay.

Treatment

Although the disease can't be cured many of the symptoms can be eased. Painkillers will help with any swelling of the joints and salivary glands, but you'll most probably have to have something stronger for the inner organs. Keeping your eyes and mouth moist by sipping liquids and using eye drops would be a big help.

Raynaud's phenomenon

Raynaud's phenomenon is a condition in which small arteries (arterioles), usually in the fingers or toes, constrict more tightly in response to exposure to cold and stress.

Raynaud's phenomenon can be seen in many healthy individuals, but is more common in people with rheumatoid arthritis (see page 53), scleroderma (see below), or as a reaction to certain drugs; for example, beta blockers.

Symptoms

Colour changes (usually white, then blue, then red) in the fingers and toes (and sometimes lips, nose and/or ear lobes) on exposure to cold. These changes may be accompanied by pain and numbness.

Treatment

If your condition is mild or moderate your doctor's first line of treatment will most probably be to ask you to make sure you keep warm, particularly around your trunk to drive warmth to the peripheries. If you're taking beta blockers or other similar medicine that constricts blood vessels he'll switch you to another medication. If this fails to improve the condition then vasodilator drugs that open up blood flow in the arterioles may be suggested.

Scleroderma

Primarily a disease that causes thickening and hardening of the skin, scleroderma in its mild and more benign form (*CREST syndrome*) is restricted to the fingers. However, it is quite likely to spread and other areas may become affected, in particular the lungs and kidneys.

Symptoms

Though best known by its thickening and hardening of the skin, scleroderma can also give rise to other symptoms such as joint pain, difficulty swallowing and shortness of breath.

Treatment

There is no cure for scleroderma, but there are a number of drugs that will ease the symptoms and exercise and physical therapy will help strengthen the body.

Polymyositis and dermatomyositis

Polymyositis is inflammation on the muscles that causes weakness. If there's an accompanying rash or other skin problems, then the disease becomes *dermatomyositis*. In certain circumstances, the lungs can also be affected.

Symptoms

Unexplained muscle weakness, usually those of the shoulder, upper arms, thighs and hips — there may also be joint pain, loss of weight and fever.

The symptoms for dermatomyositis are the same as for polymyositis with the addition of a reddish face rash and swelling around the eyes. A scaly rash may also affect the knuckles.

Treatment

The object of treatment for both diseases is to strengthen the muscles with one of the *corticosteroid drugs* called *prednisone*. (See Appendix 4, page 128.)

Treatment of the above conditions depends on their severity and the organs that are involved. Because there is an over-activity of the immune system, it's often helpful to take medications which suppress immunity such as *prednisone, azathioprine, methotrexate* and *hydroxychloroquine*. Other medications may be prescribed for relief of symptoms such as Raynaud's phenomenon, reflux (heartburn), and dryness of eyes and mouth.

Polymyalgia rheumatica and temporal arteritis

Polymyalgia rheumatica (PMR) rarely affects people under the age of 55.

Symptoms

There is inflammation in the hips and shoulders that is felt in the muscles around the neck, shoulders, upper arms, lower back, buttocks and thighs. There is often swelling in the hands and sometimes knees. It can come on overnight and cause severe pain and stiffness, making it very difficult to get out of bed. Symptoms often improve with movement. ESR and CRP are usually elevated (see page 26).

It may be associated with symptoms of a related condition called temporal arteritis (giant cell arteritis), such as headache, scalp tenderness, cramping jaw pain that comes on with chewing, and disturbance of vision. If these symptoms develop, urgent treatment may be required to prevent permanent loss of vision or stroke.

Treatment

PMR usually requires low doses of steroids, usually prednisone — higher doses are used to treat temporal arteritis. Treatment for PMR may take two to three years, but the doses of prednisone are usually quite low over most of this time.

Juvenile rheumatoid arthritis

Arthritis doesn't differentiate between the ages and, unfortunately, it can affect the young as well as adults. Juvenile rheumatoid arthritis (JRA) is an auto-immune disease where the immune system, instead of protecting the body, turns against the body and for some unknown reason causes it to destroy its own healthy tissue.

Symptoms

There are three types of JRA, each with similar though different symptoms:

Pauciarticular JRA: The most common of the three, it affects no more than four joints and, unlike RA, it isn't symmetrical, going only to one knee or one elbow. It seems to favour young pre-teen girls.

Polyarticular JRA: This attacks five or more joints, preferring the smaller ones such as fingers and toes. Like RA it is symmetrical, affecting both sets of joints.

Systemic JRA: The least common and the most problematic, it can cause trouble throughout the body, some of the symptoms being fever, inflammation of the lining of the heart and lungs, anaemia and red rash.

In all three types children will experience joint stiffness, swelling and pain, particularly after sleeping or rest. In many children the symptoms may appear only spasmodically over a period of a few months and then disappear — others less fortunate may carry the disease into adulthood.

Treatment

JRA is treated in much the same way as adult RA. (See Chapter 6, page 55.) However, it is likely that both the children and their parents may need extra emotional support.

Part three

Living with arthritis

True or false?

Copper bracelets can cure arthritis.
False
There's no evidence that wearing these bracelets helps in any way
at all, but neither do they do any harm.

Arthritis is an old people's disease.
False
There are over 1000 young New Zealanders under the age of 19
who have arthritis.

If you have arthritis you shouldn't exercise.
False
Gentle exercise is actually beneficial.

Chapter 9

The importance of exercise

!! If you haven't been physically active for many years we would strongly advise you to see your doctor before commencing any exercise programme.

It must seem rather masochistic to talk about physical exercise as part of a programme that proposes to improve the quality of life of anyone who has arthritis. But in fact the exact opposite is true; being inactive causes muscles to waste away and this puts more pressure on joints, doing further damage and increasing pain.

Many of you will be familiar with the phrase, 'Use it or lose it' — it's often called by a referee during a rugby match. Here we make the same call, but for a different reason and with a very different outcome in mind.

Unless you exercise and use your body and your muscles they'll lose their resilience and their strength and become weaker, stiffer and more painful. Exercise is not simply important, it is essential. It really is a matter of using it, or losing it! Your rheumatology team will advise you on how much and what sort of exercise you should do.

In this chapter we'd like to look at the role exercise plays in your management plan and explain why it's so relevant to your good health and wellbeing now and in the future.

What is exercise?

Exercise is any activity that gets your heart pumping, your lungs breathing, your muscles working and your joints flexing. So anything that does all that for you is exercise and will have a positive effect on both your body and your state of mind.

Specifically for people with arthritis, exercise is any activity or movement that focuses on the joints, strengthening the muscles, tendons and ligaments in order to take as much pressure as possible off the cartilage.

So, if you have arthritis, or fears that it may one day come your way, it's a matter of getting the correct balance between these two aspects of exercise and finding what is right for you.

Why should you exercise?

Until recently the medical attitude towards exercise and arthritis was to suggest that patients took it easy and stay off their feet. Unfortunately, this resulted in those with arthritis being in poorer health than people of the same age who didn't have the disease. Those with arthritis tended to be heavier, and have higher blood pressure and higher blood sugar levels. To a large extent this was because people with arthritis were conditioned to believe that inactivity was better than activity.

Fortunately, we've come a long way in the last few years and we now know that it's not good to 'take it easy and put your feet up'. We also know that there are many benefits to be enjoyed from regular exercise. Here's a few of the long-term benefits to be had:

- It's good for your heart
- It does wonders for your lungs
- It helps to keep blood pressure low
- It helps with weight control
- It promotes better balance
- It reduces stress and anxiety
- It helps you sleep better

And, it's not just physical benefits you'll enjoy — when you're exercising, your body releases a chemical called *endorphin*, which produces feelings of euphoria. It's both a painkiller and a natural form of some of the drugs that people take to get 'high' or 'turned-on'.

Once you've settled into your exercise regime you'll find three more benefits that will have quite a significant effect on your frame of mind in relation to your arthritis, namely:

- You'll be more confident and sure of yourself

- You'll have improved self-esteem
- You'll have an improved self-image

All in all we cannot stress strongly enough how important it is that you keep yourself active. There are some excellent books available detailing different exercises for different arthritis conditions, and having one at home would be well worth the expense. Alternatively, talk to your Arthritis Educator who should be able to suggest what exercises would be best for you.

The 'no pain, no gain' school of thought

Unfortunately many people think of exercise as being the regime of All Blacks and Olympic athletes — that's the 'no pain, no gain' school of exercise. That may be true for those hardy professionals, but it certainly isn't true for anyone who's just looking to keep all their parts moving as best they can.

How should you exercise?

How you get your exercise depends on a number of things: your age, your fitness, whether you want to play competitive sport or whether you just want to do the best you can for your body.

Whatever your reason, there are three basic types of exercise that should be included in any plan you make. These are:

- Cardiovascular endurance/aerobic activity
- Strength training
- Stretching/flexibility exercises

Let's have a closer look at them.

Cardiovascular endurance

Cardiovascular endurance (aerobics) activities get your heart pumping and your lungs working. This includes: walking, jogging, swimming, cycling, rowing, dancing, hopping, skipping and jumping. The value of such exertions is that they teach your heart and lungs to become more efficient in delivering oxygen to your working muscles, and when you get into the habit of doing regular cardiovascular exercises you'll soon find that you:

- Have more energy
- Lose weight
- Lower your blood pressure
- Lower your cholesterol levels
- Have a greater sense of wellbeing

!! Be careful you don't overdo it. All you need is sufficient exercise so you know that you're exerting yourself (see Gauging intensity, below). At the beginning you should try and do about 20 to 30 minutes a day, three or four times a week. As you get fitter you can increase your workout by about five minutes a month.

If you haven't been regularly exercising recently we'd recommend that you start your programme of aerobic exercises with just walking and aqua-jogging. These are easy on the joints, yet will still give you the work-out you need. Later, as you become fitter and stronger, you can progress to other aerobic activities such as cycling, dancing or swimming — and you'll find that mixing them up will be a lot more fun.

Gauging intensity

To gauge the intensity and, therefore, the value of the exercise you're doing at any given time, we use as our guide the phrase *moderate intensity*. This is the level of intensity that will give you the optimum benefit.

For example, if you're out walking with someone you should be able to talk quite easily without getting out of breath; and if you're on your own you should have no difficulty in whistling or singing to yourself. If you feel a discomfort when talking or whistling then you should slow down. On the other hand, if it's no effort at all, push yourself that little bit harder.

Strength training

The importance of strength training is that it helps develop well-toned muscles that better absorb the stresses and strains that are placed on your joints every day. If your muscles are weak, they force your joints to take the impact and this can lead to misalignment and more damage.

Strength-training exercises will improve the ability of your muscles to work efficiently over longer periods of time. We're not about to suggest that you lift heavy weights above your head. There are plenty of more comfortable ways to get your muscles working to give them strength and endurance. For instance:

- Stair climbing
- Sit-ups and push-ups
- Leg lifts
- Dancing
- Yoga (see Complementary therapies, page 36)
- Swimming
- Running

Many strength exercises will also give you a good cardiovascular work-out — you finish up with two benefits for the price of one!

Stretching

Stretching exercises to increase flexibility get you stretching, bending, reaching and twisting, and they will do wonders for your elasticity. As your muscles, ligaments, tendons and joints tend to stiffen up as you get older, making it more difficult to exercise, it's important to keep them in good shape.

Four dos and two don'ts to remember when stretching:

- Do warm-up before stretching — you should never stretch cold muscles
- Do your stretches lying on the floor so that your body's relaxed, particularly the parts you're stretching
- Do stretch slowly and carefully and hold each stretch for about 30 seconds
- Do stop if you feel pain — you could be damaging tissue

- Don't get in the habit of holding your breath when stretching — you need to get oxygen to your muscles
- Don't overdo it — let your body tell you when to stop

Warming-up and cooling-down

It's very important that you warm-up your muscles before starting to exercise. All you need is about 10 minutes, and we'd suggest you do a slow or less strenuous version of the activity you're about to do. For example, if you're planning a walk, start slowly and build up to your normal brisk pace.

It is equally important to cool-down at the end of your exercise session — all it means is you follow the reverse procedure to warming-up. For example, your brisk walk tapers down to an easy stroll. It's also a good idea to do a few gentle stretches while your muscles are warm.

Some incentives to keep you on the go

It's all too easy when you're not feeling 100 per cent and some of your old aches and pains are playing up to sit comfortably at home, do nothing and, more than likely, feel sorry for yourself. We understand only too well how easy it is to fall into that trap!

So, here are a few suggestions that may help you get up out of that chair and start you moving:

- Get someone to exercise with you; the thought of letting someone down may be all you need to get you out on a cold winter's day
- Set yourself some goals; you'll be surprised how something to aim for can focus the mind
- Keep a record of how you're exercising; you'll soon find that you'll be trying to do better one day than you did the day before
- Treat yourself to some new comfortable exercise clothes and shoes
- Play some music; listening to some of your favourite up-beat music helps your body to wake up those endorphins that make you feel good

- If your exercise is walking or running, treat yourself to a pedometer, it can become quite addictive to see how many kilometres you're eating up
- If possible exercise in the morning — you'll have a smug look on your face for the rest of the day!
- If your exercise is walking, having a dog to be responsible for will get you out on those cold days
- Don't forget that dancing is a great form of exercise and can be a lot of fun

But, the biggest incentive of all should be the fact that the profit for all the work you're doing (and the time you're putting in) is a healthier body and a more contented mind.

The green prescription

This is a government initiative set up by Sport and Recreation New Zealand (SPARC) to encourage and help New Zealanders to be more physically active. A Green Prescription is a doctor or practice nurse's written advice for a patient to be more active as part of their health self-management to increase wellbeing and minimise the need for drugs. (See their website at: <www.sparc.org.nz>.)

There are two options:

Option 1: Next time you visit your doctor or practice nurse ask them to give your details to your local Active Living coordinator, who will then get in touch with you.

Option 2: Phone 0800 22 84 83 and you'll be connected to the Active Living coordinator at your nearest regional sports trust.

!! This is a free service for everyone and is well worth the time it takes to find out about it.

What happens next?

Once you're in touch with your coordinator, your regional sports trust will offer you the following:

- Advice on the benefits of keeping active
- Help with finding suitable activities in your community
- Introductions to people with similar interests to yourself
- Help with keeping an eye on your progress
- Help with keeping your doctor advised on your progress
- A regular newsletter

When to consult your doctor

If when exercising you experience any of the following symptoms you should stop immediately and consult your doctor:

- Excessive pain or discomfort in your joints
- Changes in your normally felt symptoms
- Discomfort in your chest
- More than normal shortness of breath

!! Your exercise should require some effort but it should never be gruelling — leave that to the professionals! If you find that after a day or two of your work-out you have a few aches and pains, then you've been just a bit too energetic.

Chapter 10

Food — what's good and what's not

Many people ask us if there are any foods that will ease their arthritis. Unfortunately, gout is the only form of arthritis that can be helped by a change of diet. (See Chapter 7, page 57.) For the rest, we must answer that, other than *omega-3* and two supplements (*glucosamine* and *chondroitin,* see page 86), there is little evidence to suggest that arthritis is affected, or can be relieved by avoiding or eating any other foods.

However, that's not to say that you shouldn't give some thought to what you're eating and ask yourself the question, 'Am I doing the best I can, if not for my arthritis, then for my body?' This is a valid consideration because a healthy diet positively promotes overall good health, which will have an impact on your ability to relax and think positively. This, in turn, will help you cope with your arthritis.

We understand that sitting down to a meal you enjoy can be a source of delight and you might not relish the thought of changing the habits of a lifetime. But before you throw your hands in the air in frustration, may we offer you the following incentives? It's not as difficult as you might think and you'll certainly begin to feel much better. After a while, most people who change to a healthier diet wish they had done so much earlier. In addition:

- You may lose some weight
- Some of the new foods and recipes that are in our supermarkets today are not only healthy but also very tasty
- Get the balance right and you may reduce your risk of developing heart disease

What is a healthy diet?

First and foremost, a healthy diet is a matter of balance — it's important to balance the proteins, carbohydrates, minerals and vitamins that your body needs. Get that balance right and you'll be well on the way to having not only a healthy body, but also a much more contented mind.

Of course there are some foods you should eat and plenty that you shouldn't — or at least restrict to occasional treats — but no one's going to regiment their lives to the extent of only eating what's good for them and never touching those foods that are not so good. We all compromise a little, trade off here and there, and find a balance we can live with. In the final analysis, it all comes down to how much you care!

!! The Heart Foundation has gone to a lot of trouble on our behalf and they have identified many packaged foods that are good for the heart. That means they're good for everyone, so when you're at the supermarket keep an eye out for their friendly little tick.

Foods your body needs

To understand what constitutes a healthy diet let's first look at the basic components that make up the food we eat:

Carbohydrates: These are the starches and sugars that provide the fuel we need to run our bodies.

Carbohydrates are primarily found in vegetables, fruit, rice, cereals and sugars — and not just breakfast cereals but all products made from flour, such as bread and pasta.

Proteins: Found throughout the body in muscles, tendons, skin and blood, proteins are also the base material of our bones. Not only do proteins help our bodies grow, but also, in later life, they help us cope with the wear-and-tear of living. Dietary protein (protein that we eat) is a source of the amino acids your body needs to make its own protein.

Proteins are found in meat, poultry, fish, dairy products (not butter), eggs, tofu (soy bean curd), beans, wholegrain cereals and lentils.

Minerals: Most of us are aware that minerals are needed for our bones and teeth, but they also have many other important functions that keep our bodies working. Some of the more common minerals used by your body are: calcium, iron, magnesium, potassium, sodium and zinc.

Vitamins: These are essential for the body to work efficiently. The word vitamin comes from the words VITal AMINes. Your body can't make vitamins — they must come from the food you eat.

Fats: Fats, as well as being important building blocks for the cells of our bodies, are also the most efficient way we can consume and store energy. There are some essential fats that our bodies can't make so we must get them from the food we eat; for example, the omega-3 fatty acids found in fish and some vegetable oils.

Eat a balance of the above food groups and you'll be well on the way to having a healthy diet and, hopefully, a more positive outlook on life.

You don't have to give up that occasional after-dinner chocolate treat or the refreshing ice-cream on a sunny afternoon — just don't have them too often, and perhaps you can make up for the treat by having an extra portion or two of some good healthy fruit or vegetables. Remember, it's all a question of balance.

Foods you should be eating

One of the benefits of living in the twenty-first century is that, as far as eating is concerned, we no longer have seasons. We can buy almost any food we care to at any time we wish. In the middle of winter our supermarkets are stocked with fresh vegetables, grapefruit from South Africa, oranges from California and canned or frozen foods from all over the world. In the modern world we have no excuse to not eat well.

So what from this rich cornucopia should you put into your shopping basket? Let's have a look.

Carbohydrates

Vegetables, fruit, beans and wholegrain foods (complex carbohydrates) are at the very core of healthy eating. They are packed with fibre, minerals and naturally occurring antioxidants.

Vegetables: Freshly picked vegetables are rich in minerals, B vitamins, vitamin C, fibre and antioxidants. Slightly boiled or steamed, microwaved, stir-fried in a little olive oil, or eaten raw, they are very, very good for you. The greener, the better — so go for broccoli, cabbage, spinach, silverbeet, courgettes, peas, French beans, lettuces that aren't white — and, of course, avocados: they provide a healthy type of fat and are a great source of vitamin E.

Don't forget the other coloured vegetables: carrots, pumpkins, aubergines, red, green and yellow peppers and onions to name a few.

Frozen vegetables are fine but don't overcook them — it's best to put just a little water in the bottom of a pan and steam the vegetables with the lid on.

Fruit: Remember that old saying, 'An apple a day keeps the doctor away'? Well, it's not just apples, but all fruit — including oranges, peaches, pears, all berries, all melons, bananas, grapefruit and all those exotic fruits from the islands we now have in our supermarkets.

Dried fruit is high in fibre and potassium and has some iron. On the other hand, vitamin C is lost in the drying process and they can be loaded with concentrated sugar.

Tinned fruit will also serve you well, but only if it's canned in juice — syrup contains a large amount of sugar.

Fresh fruit juices contain vitamin C and other goodies, but can also be very high in sugar.

Wholegrains: Wheat, rice, oats, corn, barley and buckwheat are the most common wholegrain foods. These also contain many vitamins and are rich in health-preserving fibre.

As wholegrains lose much of their nutrients in milling, particularly the B vitamins and vitamin E, try and eat them whenever possible as unmilled wholegrains.

Beans: Low in fat and rich in protein, complex carbohydrates and fibre, it is best to soak dried beans overnight. The tinned variety is OK and very convenient. Check out your supermarket shelves — they have a comprehensive variety.

Pasta: It comes in many shapes and sizes — spaghetti, penne, macaroni — and makes a great base for many wholesome meals using a variety of sauces.

The Mediterranean diet

Not so much a diet but rather an approach to life, the Mediterranean diet came to prominence when it was realised that people from countries around the Mediterranean Sea — particularly Italy, Greece, France, and Spain — had an extremely low incidence of heart disease. So what was their secret?

The answer is simple — their cuisine is low in saturated fat and red meat, and high in fish and plant products, such as vegetables, fruit, pasta, grains, beans, olives and olive oil — and it's all washed down with a glass or two of red wine. Put that together with a relaxed lifestyle and it seems you've got a recipe for a pretty healthy way of life.

There are many books that give information about and recipes based on the Mediterranean diet. You'll find them in all good book shops and at your local library.

Proteins

Traditionally, eating meat, dairy products and eggs has provided our main source of protein. Though these foods contain high amounts of saturated fat they shouldn't be totally avoided, but rather eaten sparingly as they are an important source of other nutrients we need in our diet such as iron, zinc and the B-complex vitamins.

Omega-3 fatty acids

Omega-3 fatty acids are found in fish (including tinned fish and shellfish), which is an excellent alternative to meat. Small amounts of these fatty acids are also found in canola-based products; for example, linseed, walnut and wheatgerm oils. They are also found in flaxseed, which can be ground and added to bread recipes, sprinkled on hot or cold cereals or stirred into fruit or vegetable juice. Flaxseed oil is excellent in salad dressings or poured over vegetables. But you can't eat the seeds whole, as the human body cannot digest them.

!! *If you take too much omega-3 it will thin the blood — so take with caution.*

Soya beans and soy products

Soya beans and soy products are another valuable source of proteins and antioxidants and are a good alternative to meat. This includes:

Tofu: Also called soya bean curd or bean curd, tofu is made as an extract from cooked soya beans. Rich in protein, calcium and iron it is an ideal meat substitute and can be used in casseroles, stir-fries, salads, sandwiches and soups.

Tempeh: Made by fermenting soya beans which are then pressed into a cake, it is an excellent meat substitute in stir-fries.

Miso: Rich in B vitamins and protein, miso can be used in soups, sauces, dips and marinades.

Soy milk: With no saturated fat, soy milk can be used whenever a recipe calls for cow's milk.

Minerals

If you're eating a mixed diet you should be getting the minerals you need, but if you're 'salt sensitive' you might need to keep an eye on your sodium intake. The main minerals we need are:

Calcium: The most abundant mineral found in the body, any calcium deficiency will affect the bones.

Calcium mainly comes from milk and milk products such as yoghurt and cheese. Other good sources are dark green vegetables, salmon and sardines, soya beans, dried beans, peanuts and walnuts.

Magnesium: It helps you to relax and sleep better. The best natural sources are dark green vegetables, lemons, grapefruit, figs, yellow corn, almonds, nuts and seeds.

Potassium: It is found in potatoes, citrus fruits, bananas, leafy green vegetables, watercress, sunflower seeds and mint leaves.

Sodium: A mineral to be wary of; too much salt in your diet can promote high blood pressure, especially if you're 'salt sensitive'.

Sodium is found in abundance in most processed, convenience foods and particularly in salt-cured meats such as ham, bacon and corned beef. It is also found in condiments; for example, soy and chilli sauces, ketchup, and of course in those Kiwi staples, Vegemite and Marmite. Beware of hidden salt in tinned vegetables and food from your local takeaway bar.

!! In many areas of New Zealand the soils our vegetables are grown in are low in iodine so it is recommended that, when you use salt, you choose iodised salt.

Vitamins

Vitamins are organic substances that are essential for life, which can't be made by our bodies. The main vitamins we need are:

Vitamin A: One of the nutrients essential for healing wounds after surgery, vitamin A also helps to ward off infections.

Foods high in vitamin A (or its precursors, carotenens) include: sweet potatoes, carrots, pumpkin, spinach, courgettes, tomatoes, rock-melons and evaporated skim milk.

Vitamin B6: Foods rich in vitamin B6 include cabbage, wheat bran, wheat germ, wholegrain bread, brewer's yeast, cantaloupes, eggs, beef, milk, liver and kidney.

Vitamin B12: Foods rich in vitamin B12 include beef, pork, kidney, liver, cheese, eggs and milk.

Folic Acid: A form of vitamin B, folic acid is found in deep-green vegetables, carrots, avocados, beans, pumpkins, whole wheat, whole grains, melons, apricots, egg yolk and liver.

Vitamin C: Foods rich in vitamin C include fresh-picked citrus fruits, berries, green leafy vegetables, cauliflower, tomatoes, potatoes and sweet potatoes.

!! *Vitamin C levels fall when fruit is stored.*

Vitamin E: This helps in the prevention of scar tissue.

Sources of vitamin E are: vegetable oils (particularly cold-pressed virgin olive oil) and products made with them, wheat germ, whole grains, nuts, seeds, avocados and kiwifruit.

Liquids

Your body needs liquid. Next time you get thirsty, instead of reaching for a cold soft drink try some good old-fashioned water or, if you prefer, one of the many New Zealand mineral waters that are now on the market. Though not a drink, one of the many flavoured yoghurts can also work wonders.

Foods you should go easy on

We can't live without it — and for many of us — we can't live with it. Eating the following food is one of today's great dangers.

Fats

Basically there are three types of fat:

Saturated fat: This is the heart's greatest enemy. It typically comes from animal sources (the fat on beef, pork, lamb and chicken) and dairy products. Certain plant fats such as cocoa butter, palm and coconut oil also contain saturated fat.

Polyunsaturated fat: This comes from vegetable sources such as corn and sunflower, safflower and sesame seeds.

Monounsaturated fat: The friendliest fat of all, this comes from vegetable sources; for example, olives and olive oil.

Meat

When eating meat here are a few hints you should take note of:

- Processed meats, unless they're labelled 'low fat', are generally loaded with saturated fats — watch out for luncheon meats, salami, sausages, hamburgers and hot dogs
- Choose poultry rather than red meat, but avoid the skin (very fatty) and dark meat — you can't go far wrong with the white meat of a turkey
- If you're using mince, ask for low fat, or mince your own lean cuts
- On any meat you eat, cut away all the fat you can see
- Offal — liver, kidneys, brains, sweetbreads, gizzards, and hearts — are packed full of saturated fats and should be restricted for use as occasional treats
- Eat smaller portions

Dairy products

Most dairy products are loaded with saturated fat and you should be wary of them. This includes:

Butter: It is full of saturated fat and the alternative, margarine, is full of trans-fatty acids (see page 85), so what can you do? Fortunately, there are now spreads that have been enriched with plant sterols and stanols, which provide a safe alternative to butter and margarine.

!! Sterols and stanols are naturally occurring components of all plants. Mainly found in vegetable oils, traces are also found in fruit and vegetables.

Cheese, cream, milk: These are all high in saturated fats. Hard cheeses generally have lower levels than soft cheeses, and low-fat milk is OK. Unless it is labelled low fat, ice-cream should be on your 'only as a treat' list. Yoghurt is great for you.

Chocolate: Not only is it made with full-fat milk but also cocoa butter, which is one of the plant sources of saturated fat. Put this on your 'only as a treat' list.

Trans-fatty acids and hydrogenation

The process of making shortening and margarine, whereby liquid vegetable oils are converted to being either solid or semi-solid, is called *hydrogenation*. The resulting products are called *trans-fatty acids*.

Though derived from good vegetable oils, trans-fatty acids act more like saturated fat as they increase the levels of heart-damaging cholesterol.

Trans-fatty acids increase the shelf-life of commercially prepared foods and can be found in many processed convenience foods, such as potato chips, biscuits and cake mixes.

Eggs

Eggs used to be thought of as quite dangerous but now, if eaten in moderation, are considered a healthy food choice.

The villain of the egg is the yolk, so if you're partial to omelettes or scrambled eggs, use one whole egg and one egg white instead of two whole eggs. You might also consider a similar technique in any recipe that doesn't require too many eggs.

!! Beware of convenience, processed, tinned and fast foods — they generally contain high levels of sodium.

Those extra kilos

For many people when they think they are overweight, they think of it in terms of their appearance or how badly their clothes seem to fit. Now and again, they may consider that perhaps they should be doing something about it.

Well, we'd like to suggest another way of looking at being overweight. If you're carrying more kilos than you should be for your body size, you'll be subjecting those joints that allow you to stand, sit, bend and walk — your hips, knees and ankles — to a force far greater than your overall weight. For example, when you step on the scales the needle shoots up to 100 kg before settling back to 70 kg. If you jump on the scales, it might shoot up to 200 kg — this is the momentary force through the joints which the cartilage must be able to withstand. The more you weigh, the greater this momentary force will be. Every time you take a step or get up out of a chair, you're putting even more force on to your joints.

If you have arthritis one of your greatest enemies is being overweight and we cannot stress strongly enough how important it is that you do everything in your power to shed any excess kilos and keep your weight under control.

Supplements

Supplements are big business nowadays and can be bought from health shops, chemists and even supermarkets. However, the only supplements that have been shown to be of benefit if you have arthritis are:

Glucosamine and chondroitin: These will help reduce the pain of osteoarthritis. However, recent studies have cast doubt on previous research findings that showed a benefit for these supplements — it appears that some brands work and others don't.

Fish oil, omega-3: These help reduce inflammation and inflammatory arthritis. (See also page 81.)

!! If you wish to take any other supplements we would advise you to first discuss it with your doctor or arthritis nurse.

Body Mass index

Body mass index (BMI) is a measure of weight adjusted for height and is calculated by dividing a person's weight (in kilograms) by their height (in metres) squared.

The algebraic formula for this is:

$$BMI = \frac{kg}{m^2}$$

BMI is used to classify men and women between the ages of 18 and 65 as overweight and obese. It is an indicator to determine if those extra kilos you're carrying place you at risk of developing health problems. In New Zealand, adults are defined as overweight if their BMI is 25.0–29.9 and obese if BMI is 30.0 or more.

Ethnicity can alter the BMI, and for Maori and Pacific adults overweight is defined as a BMI of 26.0–31.9 and obesity as BMI 32.0 or more.

Don't worry if you can't work it out. Your doctor or arthritis educator will have a chart and will figure it out for you. There is also a BMI calculator online at <www.halls.md/body-mass-index/bmi.htm>

However, BMI has limitations for determining whether your weight is ideal or not as it cannot distinguish lean muscle and body fat. If you have any concerns about your weight, discuss them with your doctor or arthritis educator on your next visit.

Chapter 11

Getting through the days

In Chapter 3 we talked about the gate theory of pain (see page 33) and suggested that 'gates' existed along our nerve pathways, which could, depending on certain conditions, open or close and thereby control the strength of the pain messages that we feel.

Scientists have learned that one of the influential 'controllers' of these gates is our state of mind and that the more stressed or angry we are, the more the gates open and the more pain we feel.

The irony here, of course, is that it's the condition itself — the arthritis — and the pain or discomfort that goes with it that causes our negative state of mind and those feelings of stress and anger. Yet we've got a life to live — family responsibilities, a wage to be earned, household work to be done, pets to care for, hobbies and a social life to enjoy. Sometimes the stress of just getting through a day puts such a strain on us that it's all too easy to get angry — and so the 'gates' open up and more pain gets through and we get angrier and more stressed. It's a vicious cycle.

So is there anything you can do to break the cycle and hold back those demons of anger and stress? Fortunately, we've learned much about the relationship between body and mind in recent years and for most people the answer is an emphatic, 'Yes, there certainly is!'

The first thing to do is understand your condition and accept it. It's only through understanding and acceptance of your arthritis that you can begin to control it, rather than letting it control you. Learning about stress and how you respond to it will help you fight against those feelings of anger that can so often flare up when you encounter a stressful situation.

Stress

Stress is your body's response to situations that frighten, scare or challenge you. You're more than likely going to become stressed if you are faced with change. The important thing to understand is that it's not what happens to you that causes your stress, but rather how you react to what happens.

And it's important to realise that not all stress comes from negative situations. Going on a holiday or getting married are both happy events, but both carry within them elements of stress and the potential for individuals to become stressed.

Managing stress

The secret to managing stress is to focus on how you react to a stressful situation and not on the situation itself. Here are some suggestions:

- Identify the situations that are likely to cause you to become stressed and either avoid them or learn how to cope with them
- Take time to smell the roses — stress thrives in those who are always in a hurry (see The Type-A personality, page 91)
- Recognise the signs — the more you let stress build up the harder it is to stop
- Be organised — you'll be able to anticipate and avoid those stressful situations that you haven't yet learned to control
- Remember the old adage, 'To be forewarned is to be forearmed'
- Make sure you have quality time for yourself and you get plenty of rest — tiredness can play havoc with your perceptions
- Keep things in proportion — if you miss a bus, chances are there'll be another one along soon
- Be open with others — it will help them understand you and your needs
- Don't aim your expectations so high that they're unattainable — don't most of us measure our contentment by the difference between our expectations and reality?
- Always look on the bright side; the glass is half full not half empty, isn't it?

- It's better to be concerned about things rather than worried; champions win games because they concern themselves with the game, not because they worry about its outcome

Pacing yourself

One of the characteristics of arthritis is that you have good days and bad days and this can very easily become a trap for anyone who's only recently been diagnosed as having arthritis and put on medication. Imagine, you've been experiencing pain for maybe months and here you are, the medicine's kicking in, the pain has eased and suddenly you're back for a whole day in that garden that's been so badly neglected for so long. That's really not a good idea — the garden may look better, but it's doubtful you will!

It's all a matter of pacing yourself and that means you're going to have to change your mindset and how you do things. Of course, you can still do your favourite activities but you need to do them in a different way; for example, spend only half a day in the garden, and then only if you've made sure that you've taken adequate pain relief and sufficient anti-inflammatory protection.

Having arthritis puts you on a huge learning curve and if you take the time and make the effort, you're going to get to know yourself extremely well. Then, with time, it will be your body, nothing else, that tells you how long you should spend in the garden. You are the only person who knows how your body works and by listening to it you will learn to pace yourself.

Stressful moments

Here are some of the more common situations that are almost guaranteed to create stress. Knowing about them (if possible) allows you to plan to minimise your stressful responses:

- Death of a loved one
- Marital break-up
- Losing a job
- Changing jobs
- Birth of a child
- Marital reconciliation
- Retirement
- Going on holiday

The Type-A personality

Whether we like it or not, in the modern world we put a high value on acquiring material possessions and, generally, we hold those who succeed in such endeavours in high esteem. Success is all important and the criterion for success has become the acquisition of 'things'.

Now, that's not a bad thing in itself. Why shouldn't we enjoy the comforts of the modern world? Unfortunately, in the scramble for success many people have developed a form of behaviour that creates a personality type that is driven by an excessively competitive drive — what we call a Type-A personality. Here are some of the indications that point to a Type-A personality:

- Having a somewhat aggressive and hostile nature
- Tending to always be tense and unable to relax
- Always running out of time
- Always being in a hurry with somewhere to go or someone to see
- Having a tendency to be selfish — people who are only interested in talking about things that relate to themselves
- Being impatient and easily bored
- Having a habit of often finishing other people's sentences
- Feeling guilty when not 'doing' something
- Playing games to win, not just for the fun of it

If you recognise yourself as having some of the above characteristics, you may well be a Type-A personality and this could be contributing to your pain levels. It's unlikely that you're going to change overnight, but there's much that you can do to lessen the stress that is impacting on your arthritis.

Take a close look at the points above that apply to you, and from now on make a conscious effort to turn every one of them around. So, slow down and treat yourself to some time in which to laugh and have some fun. Pick more daisies!

- Selling a house
- Financial problems
- Divorce

- Buying a house
- Winning Lotto
- Marriage

Of course, there are many other personal situations that send the stress barometer flying through the roof, especially for anyone with a condition such as arthritis that is with you each and every day.

!! *Remember, you may not be able to change the things that give you stress, but you can change your attitudes and responses by reshaping your view of them.*

Anger

If you look up the word 'anger' in a Thesaurus you'll find it coupled with words like *resentment, displeasure, discontent* and *irritation.* Ring a bell? If you have arthritis then surely these are words you're familiar with and understand only too well. But, did you know that these words can also be attributed to the Type-A personality we've described — those competitive individuals who are always on the run, hate to waste time, can't sit still for a moment and are always racing against the clock.

If you're a Type-A personality and you have arthritis, your 'pain gates' are most likely going to open more often than they need to because you're inclined to feel *displeased, discontented* and *irritated* by many things other than your arthritis.

So what should you do? The answer to that question, whatever type of personality you are, lies in your understanding of yourself, accepting who you are and that, unless you're comfortable with your current situation, there needs to be some changes.

Many of the suggestions we made for coping with stress also apply to managing anger and frustration, so have another look at them. You might find the following useful as well:

- Slow down — you may be in a hurry, but the world isn't

- Give your priorities a thought and find out just what's important to you and, more importantly, what's not — if you don't clean the car this weekend, is that really such a disaster?

- Have some fun and remember to include all those people you care for and love

- Share your frustrations — a problem shared is a problem halved

- And most important of all, there are things in your life that you can't change, so do try and accept them — being angry can only make things worse

Depression

Because of the intrusive nature of arthritis many people, some for the first time in their lives, get to know the full meaning of the word depression, that all-invading, frightening, black feeling that when it's with you, you truly believe you'll never be able to escape. You're for ever tired, you can't sleep, you become irritable. That leads to stress and all of a sudden you're angry — all the conditions that are right for opening those 'pain gates'.

Unfortunately, it's difficult to overcome depression as it comes at you from two fronts:

Physically: Depression makes you tired and inactive and for many people their response is to stay in bed, sometimes for a day, sometimes for much longer. Such inactivity, over time, leads to a general decline of fitness — muscles begin to weaken, joints start to stiffen — the two conditions which can, and often do, lead to increased pain.

Mentally: Depression lowers the levels of your body's natural pain-killer — endorphins, and your pain levels go up a notch or two.

So you find yourself in the strange situation where your pain causes you to be depressed and your resulting depression causes you more pain.

As an indication that you are experiencing clinically significant depression you will show at least one of the following characteristics:

- Prolonged and strong feelings of depression which include sadness, dejection, rejection and other such feelings of worthlessness

- Low activity levels — you don't seem to be doing much and you're beginning to let things you normally do slide

- A tendency to see life as making overwhelming demands

on you and placing insurmountable problems in your way

- Feeling a sense of hopelessness about the future and that things are never going to get better
- Sleeping difficulties — either sleeping too much or not sleeping at all
- Having constant feelings of fatigue and a lack of enthusiasm or energy

!! There are varying degrees of depression and not everyone who is depressed shows all the above characteristics. But if one or more apply to you we would strongly advise that you see your doctor and discuss the matter with him.

Getting a good night's sleep

It's no joy lying in bed at night, in pain, tossing and turning and hoping desperately that you'll shut your eyes and it'll be morning. It seems that as we get older, sleep eludes us and what was once the comfortable refuge of our bed becomes our own torture chamber.

If these feelings are familiar to you the very first thing to do is to talk to your doctor. In addition to whatever he suggests, we'd like to offer the following advice:

- Have your last drink of tea, coffee or cocoa around about six in the evening — they contain caffeine which is a stimulant and will most probably keep you awake
- Before going to bed, and not in or on the bed, treat yourself to about an hour of quiet relaxation; read a book, listen to music or a relaxation tape or just simply meditate — what you don't want to do is to have serious discussions solving the problems of the world, because stimulating the mind doesn't help you sleep
- Try a long soak in a hot bath, particularly on a cold winter's night
- Try and set your body's internal clock by going to bed and getting up at the same time each day, even on weekends

- Check that your mattress and pillows are as comfortable as they can be — have a chat to your occupational therapist

- You may find that a quiet walk in the evening will help, but we stress it must be no more than a gentle stroll

- Is your bedroom as dark and as quiet as it could be? A relaxation tape or CD playing quietly in the background may help, but make sure it's on 'repeat mode' as the silence when it stops could well wake you

- Try out a 'white noise machine' that will give out a multi-frequency sound, like a WHOOSH that supposedly relaxes you and blocks out all other noises

Keep your bed for sleeping and sex; it's not for reading, watching television, talking to a friend on the phone, eating, writing letters or any other activity. It is your own private, personal island and you should treat it as such.

Your occupational therapist

An occupational therapist (OT) will work with you on four different levels helping you learn the easiest and most efficient way to get through your day:

Level 1: Together you will look at the things you have to do on a daily basis and devise the easiest ways for you to do them; e.g. getting dressed, getting you looking good, preparing meals, eating, getting around, going shopping, doing the housework and going to work.

Level 2: Your OT will tell you about all the special labour-saving devices that are available and will recommend those that will make your life easier.

Level 3: Your OT will help you draw up your self-management plan.

Level 4: Most importantly, your OT will show you how to conserve your energy. We all only have so much energy and when that runs out, just like a motor car that runs out of petrol, we come to a full stop.

Some of the things you'll be looking at are:

- How best to plan ahead: What shortcuts can you find? What things can be done at the same time?

- How to prioritise things and make sure you get the important things done first

- How to pace yourself and manage the balancing act between being active and resting

Remember, your occupational therapist is a trained professional who's there to help you understand the physical limitations that your conditions place on you and how you can best overcome them. If you have any questions, don't hesitate to ask them.

Making things easy

You'll be surprised when you see the list of gadgets that are available to make your life that little bit easier:

- Doorknob and key turners
- Shower seats
- Voice-activated computers
- Automatic jar openers
- Toothpaste tube squeezers
- Stretch shoe laces
- Raised toilet seats
- Voice-activated telephones
- Long-handled comb
- Plastic bag openers
- Easy-pull sock aid
- Non-slip grips for cups
- Easy-hold cups and glasses
- Soap and lotion applicators

These and other helpful aids are available from a number of suppliers — talk to your arthritis educator.

Arthritis, sex and intimacy

Having arthritis and trying to manage your pain, medication and your physical limitations can only too often lead to a decline in both your self-image and your sexual drive. You may feel inadequate. Attempts at intercourse may turn to disaster as each of you is aware of the possibility of pain: lubrication can stop, an erection can disappear and an intimate romantic encounter becomes another frustrating attempt at physically expressing your sexuality.

What can you do? Fortunately, there is an answer: don't think of 'intercourse' but rather think in terms of 'intimacy'. Sex doesn't necessarily have to be coital and penetrative; it can be many other things. Gently stroking, kissing and caressing are quite wondrous ways of expressing your sexuality and showing the care and love you have for each other.

With time and having no predetermined standard of performance to achieve, perhaps intercourse will be possible. On the other hand, you may enjoy a new-found intimacy and want no more than that.

How to build a mutually pleasing sexual relationship

Most book shops and libraries have a whole range of books on sexual relationships and we strongly recommend that you have a look and choose one that suits your needs. Here we offer a few suggestions to help you and your partner build a mutually pleasing sexual relationship:

- Talk about your feelings, your fears and your sexual needs — New Zealand men are not the best at opening themselves up so it might be up to the woman to take the initiative

- Even though you may be the one with arthritis, your partner is going through much the same mental strain as you

- While spontaeous sex can be exciting and explosive so too can planned sex: choose in advance an evening when neither of you is going to be too tired — don't be shy, talk about it beforehand and share your expectations with each other, listen to each other

- Select a warm room, have some of your favourite music playing, and make sure the lighting isn't so bright that it shows up imperfections

- Have a bath (separately), don't forget the bath salts and a little perfume or aftershave

- Dress in something revealing and what the prudish might call 'naughty'

Sharing your problems

Many people find that one of the most difficult aspects of having arthritis, as with many other medical conditions, is how to handle their sexuality. As well as the psychological impact of the disease there is, for some, what they see as the stigma of physical deformity that accompanies many forms of arthritis.

So, if you are faced with such difficulties, what is the best way to overcome them? Unfortunately, there's no single or simple answer we can offer except to say that however you see the problem, there is an answer and it will inevitably lie in your sharing the problem with your partner. If for any reason you find this impossible, confide in a friend or another family member; and if you don't feel able to do this, ask your doctor or arthritis educator to put you in touch with a professional counsellor.

How do you manage if you're not in a relationship?

We should first point out that though sexual chemistry is important, most lasting relationships evolve over time and depend upon shared interests rather than the initial physical attraction.

People meet each other in many different ways — through friends, work, social clubs and, more and more nowadays, through the internet. It's important that, no matter how you feel, you should not lose contact with the outside world — there's someone out there who's looking for you.

Who can help?

First and foremost, talk with your arthritis educator through Arthritis New Zealand: Freephone 0800 663 463.

For the young at heart Arthritis New Zealand runs a special group called YAP (Young arthritis persons). They're well worth a call, also on: Freephone 0800 663 463.

The Arthritis Research Campaign in the UK has an excellent website: <www.arc.org.uk>. Click on 'Site Index' then 'Sexuality and arthritis'.

Arthritis support groups

For many years now people with arthritis have been getting together outside the hospital environment and establishing support groups for themselves. Some are run by the members themselves, others by health professionals (doctors, nurses, occupational therapists or social workers). The objectives of each group vary greatly; some are based on education while others offer emotional support and somewhere to share experiences.

Some groups are specifically for a single type of arthritis, such as osteoarthritis or rheumatoid arthritis; others are a catch-all for all forms of arthritis.

If you're thinking of joining a support group we'd suggest you shop around and find one that suits you. Don't make a decision on one visit alone; try it at least twice because, just like individuals, groups can have good days and bad days. Here are some reasons to join a support group:

- It'll get you out of the house and interacting with other people who share similar conditions and will understand how you feel
- Education — you'll learn about your condition
- Through sharing you'll learn how other people solve their own similar problems
- There'll be ideas on how to cope with situations that may be problematic for you
- Encouragement — you'll meet people whose arthritis is more advanced than yours and see that they're living full and productive lives

!! To find a support group in your area contact Arthritis New Zealand on: Freephone 0800 663 463.

Chapter 12

The power of the mind

So far we've mostly talked about the medical aspects of arthritis: what the disease is; what the treatment options are; how pain affects you; the stress you're likely to be under; the anger you may feel; and the depression that's likely to grow out of that stress and anger. It's pretty heavy stuff and you must be wondering if there's anything positive that can be said about having arthritis. Or is this all you have to look forward to in the future?

The outcome for you is going to depend on you and the way you choose to approach the future. There are thousands of people in New Zealand who live with arthritis, the vast majority of whom have accepted their condition and live happy fulfilled lives. They're not supermen or superwomen, just ordinary people who happen to have an illness that restricts the activities they're able to enjoy.

Of course the key word here is 'acceptance': if you're to move forward in a positive manner you must, first and foremost, accept that your arthritis is something that's a reality and you're not going to wake up one morning and find that it's gone and all is well with the world! You've got to get over the fact that there are some things that you just can't change, however much you might want to. Once you reach that acceptance, not just on the surface but deep down in your heart, only then can you begin to start thinking positively about your condition and how you're going to build yourself a better life around it.

Did you know?

The famous French painter Pierre-Auguste Renoir had rheumatoid arthritis and in his later years had to have his paint brushes tied to his hands. When he couldn't paint any more he took up sculpture!

Positive thinking

The frustrating thing about having a mind of our own is that we sometimes completely forget we have one, and the older we get the more we tend to ignore it. Somehow, we seem to overlook the fact that we have the ability to harness this great friend and ally to help us take control of our attitudes and emotions.

If we allow the problems of our arthritis to constantly dominate our thinking, then those thoughts will feed into our subconscious and act as confirmation of our negativity, and our problems will seem magnified. However, if we work together with our minds and feed them thoughts of wellbeing, even if we don't feel all that well, then the power of our minds will follow those positive thoughts and our problems will seem less important.

For example, if you wake up one morning and, for some perverse reason, you tell yourself you're going to be miserable all day and you keep repeating that message to yourself, your family and friends, it's not difficult to imagine that by about lunchtime you're going to be a very unhappy person indeed!

The secret is in knowing and believing that there is a powerful link between your mind and your body, and that you have the power to influence and strengthen that link so that your subconscious mind will make your (positive) thoughts a reality. By working together with this tremendous positive force it's possible to modify your reality. It needs practice — practice, more practice and even more practice — but it is possible and you'll find that it's well worth the effort.

Here are some suggestions to get you started:

- Think of things as right, good and happy rather than wrong, bad and sad
- Don't feel sorry for yourself — although this is not always easy, remember that there are plenty of people who'd exchange places with you instantly
- Be creative in your thinking — dismiss negative thoughts from your mind and replace them with positive ones
- Repeat positive thoughts to yourself throughout the day — try writing them down
- If you daydream make sure the dreams are happy ones —

have you ever heard of anyone dreaming of losing the lottery?

- Be positive in your thinking — the bottle should be half full rather than half empty
- Don't worry about things you have no control over

!! *Get it right and you'll discover that even unexpected dark clouds can sometimes have quite wonderful silver linings.*

The spirit within

In learning to control your mind and encourage it towards steadily improving your quality of life through positive thoughts and feelings, you call on that intangible part of yourself that is the very fundamental, emotional and activating principle of your being — your 'spirit'.

Deep inside all of us, under many layers of conditioning, is this force of life that animates our bodies and governs our beliefs and our behaviour. Some of us express this spirit in the celebration of a religion, promoting times of quiet, meditation and prayer. For others, spirituality is expressed in the celebration of nature — flowers, trees, the waters of rivers, the sounds of birds and the cool feel of a gentle breeze. Great musicians, writers, poets and painters find their spiritual satisfaction in their artistic expression. And, if one is cynical, you might say that in recent times the celebration of this spirit is to be found in the pursuit of material 'things'.

However you choose to acknowledge this force of life, this spirit, it is part of your being and has a strong influence on your ability to positively influence your mind and your life. Learn about it and understand it for, in so doing, you will positively affect your way of thinking and you will be all the richer for it. Your spirit links you to a power far greater than any power you consciously possess and if you neglect it you will be infinitely the poorer.

You are more than your arthritis

Too many people, when told that their arthritis has been confirmed, seem totally overcome and allow it to take control of their lives. They seem to forget that they're still the same person they were before and that, although there are probably things they can no longer do, they can still laugh when there's humour, cry when things are sad, love and be loved, watch their children and grandchildren grow into adults, enjoy a beautiful sunset or a good film. Indeed, all those things they've been doing and enjoying all their lives — most of them are still there to be enjoyed.

The message to remember from this is that you are far more than your arthritis and you should keep this at the forefront of your mind.

The grieving process

Being told that you have a chronic illness and that you must live with it for the rest of your life can, if you let it, be the beginning of a life-long grieving process.

Most grieving processes are about loss; if you have arthritis the loss that you're grieving isn't what you'd experience on losing a loved one or a friend, but rather it's the feeling of loss of yourself, of what you can no longer be or do or have. It can be the loss of your former good health, the loss of being able to have a proper night's sleep, the loss of self-image or, possibly, the loss of what can no longer be achieved in the future. And so you grieve.

But like all loss, you will eventually come to terms with it. With the help and encouragement of family and friends and the medical professionals you'll soon realise that you are far more than your arthritis, and once you get the past into perspective, you'll soon find meaning in the present and hope for the future.

Chapter 13

Travelling with arthritis

If you have arthritis and your condition is stable, then you should have no worries about travelling. Listed below are a few hints that we hope will make your travelling safer and more enjoyable.

Travelling by plane

Drugs: Take sufficient medicine to last you the whole trip. In fact, we recommend that you also take a spare set of medicines in case one gets lost, or you end up staying longer than planned. Have one set in your hand luggage, the other packed in your suitcase. Just to be on the safe side, keep a list of the medication you're on with your travel documents — generic and brand names.

Medical history: Before you leave, it might pay you, depending on your condition, to get a letter from your doctor with details of your arthritis history and keep it with you on your trip.

Time zones: If you're changing time zones, talk it over with your doctor to see how it will affect the medication you're on. It's probably best to travel using your home time zone, and then make any changes to your medication time on your arrival. But do get some advice.

Seating: When making your booking ask for an aisle seat, this will enable you to get in and out more easily.

Exercise: To ease joint stiffness on long journeys walk up and down the aisle every hour or so and, if you can find the space, do a few stretching exercises

Stopovers: Be open with your travel agent about your condition and discuss the best routes to take. For example, unless you're staying overnight, stopovers in the USA can be quite long and arduous, so to get to Europe the Asian alternative may be easier on both body and mind.

Luggage: Be careful and selective in what you pack — most passengers take far too many clothes and use only a few. Use luggage that is easy to move around, preferably with wheels. Always carry your documents, money and other valuable belongings with you in your hand luggage.

Avoid rushing: Plan to arrive at the airport early rather than at the last minute — remember traffic is often unpredictable. Avoid carrying heavy suitcases: use trolleys as much as you can or, alternatively, use a porter. (You'll be amazed how quickly they can take you to the top of the queue!) Try to avoid tight airline connections — there will always be another plane (and usually, though not always, the airline will put you up in a hotel if you miss a connecting flight).

Clothes: Wear comfortable, loose clothes while travelling — it's not a fashion parade. If you feel cold ask for a blanket — all planes carry them. Find out what the weather is likely to be at your destination, and have appropriate clothing in your hand luggage.

Air pressure: Most planes are pressurised and for most of us this doesn't present a problem. However, if you have an airway disease, such as emphysema or bronchitis, you should discuss this with both your doctor and the airline.

Meals: Airline food is reasonably harmless, although it can often pay you to order low-fat, low-salt meals when you're making your reservations as these are generally of a higher quality and often tastier than meals provided for other passengers.

If you should feel unwell during the trip: Don't be shy — tell one of your flight attendants, they are very well trained and equipped for emergencies and they'll also know if there's a doctor or nurse on board who can help.

Wheelchairs: Most modern airports have long walks to and from the planes and you may well find such a distance difficult. Not to worry — tell somebody at the check-in (or on the plane before you land) that you would like some assistance and a wheelchair will always be provided. This also usually results in your getting some VIP treatment as well!

Deep vein thrombosis (DVT)

Commonly known as DVT or economy class syndrome, long-distance airline travel can cause clots to form in the legs and sometimes these can break off and block the arteries leading to the lungs (*pulmonary embolism*). This is usually due to a combination of dehydration and lack of movement. However, there are a few simple precautions you can take to minimise the risk:

- Reduce the length of your flights by planning stopovers whenever possible
- Wear comfortable shoes and clothes
- Drink plenty of water
- A little alcohol with your meal is fine but be careful as alcohol taken in planes can cause dehydration
- Choose a seat on the aisle and every now and again get up and walk a little
- Stretch your legs forward as much as you can when resting, as it is bending at the knees and hips that causes the blood to flow less freely
- Don't cross your legs
- Wear supportive stockings

Travelling by car

The secret to long car journeys is to arrange your trip so that you have plenty of stops when you can get out and move about. When starting the journey again, you may want to change places and sit in one of the other seats.

Chapter 14

Pregnancy and arthritis

Just because someone has arthritis doesn't mean that they can't, or shouldn't, have children. However, given that inflammatory arthritis commonly affects women of childbearing years, it's not uncommon for rheumatologists to be involved in the care of women with arthritis who wish to become pregnant, are currently pregnant or have recently had a baby.

!! If you have arthritis and wish to start a family it is imperative that you discuss the idea with your rheumatologist at least six months before conception. This applies to both men and women. Many arthritis medications have the potential to cause harm to a developing baby and cannot be used during pregnancy.

There are, of course, many issues to be assessed and discussed, but it should be stressed that arthritis and related conditions are seldom a barrier to having children. Let's look at some of the important issues.

The effect of arthritis on fertility

Arthritis does not usually affect the ability to conceive. Though women with arthritis tend to have smaller families than non-arthritic women, this is usually by choice, or because of circumstances of their health that required them to avoid becoming pregnant, rather than their inability to get pregnant.

The effect of arthritis on pregnancy

It's unlikely that arthritis will interfere with your pregnancy except in two cases:

- If you have *anti-phospholipid syndrome* (see Appendix 1, page 111)
- If you have severe *scleroderma* (see Appendix 1, page 113)

The effect of pregnancy on arthritis

The effect of pregnancy on arthritis will vary from person to person, though there are two instances worth mentioning:

- Rheumatoid arthritis usually goes into remission in early pregnancy and flares up again either after delivery or when breast-feeding stops
- Severe lupus with kidney involvement can be made worse by pregnancy

Your helpful friends

If you're planning to start a family we would suggest that after you've talked to your rheumatologist and doctor you get in touch with both your local physiotherapist and occupational therapist. They'll help you manage your pregnancy, maintain your muscle tone and make sure you keep up your strength.

After your baby's been born they'll show you different ways of holding, lifting and bathing your baby with the minimum of effort and, should you need them, they'll help you find the right splints and gadgets that will make your life that much easier. Also, should a flare occur both therapists will be of great help assisting you to care for your newborn treasure.

If you go to antenatal classes you need to let the health professionals know about your condition so that they're aware of it and can meet any special needs you may have.

If you haven't already done so, you may want to contact Arthritis New Zealand who'll advise you through your pregnancy and possibly put you in touch with other women who have had arthritis and given birth. A shared experience can be both helpful and beneficial. (See Appendix 2, page 115.)

The usual problems of pregnancy such as backache, sciatica and carpal tunnel syndrome apply to pregnant women with arthritis as much as to anyone, though the symptoms are often somewhat worse.

The effect of medication on pregnancy

Some drugs should be avoided at all costs during pregnancy. These include:

- methotrexate
- D-penicillamine
- leflunomide
- gold injections
- cyclophosphamide

If you're taking any of the above medications and you wish to start a family it is imperative that you discuss this with your rheumatologist or doctor at least six months before conception. Methotrexate should be avoided by both men and women at the time of, and for three months before, insemination.

Sulphasalazine, hydroxychloroquine and low-dose prednisone are regarded as safe in pregnancy. However, sulphasalazine can lower the sperm count in men.

Paracetamol is safe during pregnancy.

Joint injections are safe during pregnancy.

Non-steroidal anti-inflammatory drugs (NSAIDs) can be used in the first and second trimesters, but should be avoided in the third trimester. However, there is evidence of a slightly increased risk of miscarriage in women taking NSAIDs at the time of conception.

NSAIDs may temporarily decrease fertility, but the effect is slight, so DO NOT rely on this as a contraceptive. If you're having difficulty getting pregnant it might be worth coming off your NSAID.

The effect of medication on breast-feeding

If you need to restart disease-modifying anti-rheumatic drugs after delivery (see Appendix 4, page 129), it is usually best to wean your baby first.

Fast-acting NSAIDs can be used if they are taken immediately after breast-feeding. This will mean that the dose in the milk will be low by the time you feed your baby again. Don't exceed the recommended maximum daily dose — you don't have to take the NSAID after every breast-feed.

Paracetamol is safe while breast-feeding.

Joint injections are safe while breast-feeding.

!! *Always consult your doctor before starting or restarting any medication during pregnancy or when breast-feeding.*

The effect of parenthood on arthritis

Frequent night-time feeds can deprive you of the sleep you need and could well worsen your overall pain levels. Share the duties with your spouse/partner. This is easy to do if you are bottle-feeding, but if you are breast-feeding you may want to try letting your partner bottle-feed using expressed milk.

Take extra rest during the day while your baby is asleep and get help with the housework.

Caring for a baby is physically demanding, especially on the hands, wrists, elbows, shoulders and back. Use wrist splints, and when you're lifting remember to lift with your knees. (See also Your helpful friends, page 108.)

Appendix 1:
Glossary of terms

Acupressure: A form of Asian medicine similar to acupuncture (see below) that uses fingers and hands rather than needles. Also called *shiatsu*.

Acupuncture: A Chinese practice of inserting needles to balance the energy flow in the body.

Acute pain: Pain that has developed recently.

Ankylosing: Joining together, as in Ankylosing spondylitis, which means literally 'inflammation causing joining together of bones in the spine'.

Anti-phospholipid syndrome: Antibodies in the blood that can cause clots and miscarriage. These clots can block blood vessels causing pulmonary embolism and stroke.

Aromatherapy: Practitioners of this believe that there are certain scents and aromas that can help the healing process.

Arthritis: Literally 'inflamed joints', but it describes any disease of the joints.

Arthrodesis: Fusion of a joint.

Arthroplasty: Joint surgery, usually replacement.

Arthroscopy: Examination of the inside of a joint through an inserted 'telescope'.

Auto-immune disease: When your immune system, which is normally meant to fight infection, turns against your own body tissue.

Biomechanics: The study of the movement in relation to each other of bones, joints, muscles, tendons and ligaments.

Bursitis: Inflammation of a lubricating pad between musculoskeletal structures, e.g. a tendon and a bone.

Cartilage: The smooth, hard point of contact between bones inside a joint.

Chondroitin sulphate: A supplement that may ease the symptoms of osteoarthritis.

Chronic pain: Pain that has been present for some time or that keeps recurring.

Complementary medicine: Any treatment undertaken in conjunction with your conventional medical care and which you find eases your pain or discomfort.

Corticosteroids: Anti-inflammatory drugs that mimic the effects of the natural hormone cortisol.

Dermatomyositis: An auto-immune inflammatory disease of muscle and skin.

Discoid lupus erythematosus: A form of lupus with patches of rash as the main symptom.

DMARDs: Disease modifying anti-rheumatic drugs which reduce the damage to joints.

Flares: Episodes of worsening of inflammation, usually in more than one joint, in a patient whose disease had been under control.

Glucosamine: A substance derived from natural sources that may reduce the symptoms of osteoarthritis.

Gout: An inflammatory disease of the joints and soft tissues caused by deposition of needle-shaped uric acid crystals.

Immunosuppressants: Drugs that dampen inflammation caused by overactivity of the immune system.

Joints: The junctions between bones that allow smooth movement of one bone in relation to another.

Juvenile arthritis (sometimes labelled JIA or RCA): Arthritis of various forms that develops in childhood and early adolescence.

Ligaments: Tough bands of fibrous tissue that join bones to each other.

NSAIDs: Non-steroidal anti-inflammatory drugs that relieve the symptoms of inflammation without having corticosteroid effects.

Occupational therapist: A health professional trained to assess and help patients manage the practical aspects of daily life.

Omega-3 fatty acids: Fats and oils derived from fish and plants that reduce inflammation if they make up a significant component of the daily fat intake.

Orthopaedic surgeon: A surgeon specialising in bones and joints.

Osteoarthritis: A form of arthritis in which cartilage degrades, resulting in changes to the bone around the affected joint(s).

Physiotherapist: A health professional who uses physical treatments and exercise to treat musculoskeletal disorders.

Psoriatic arthritis: An inflammatory arthritis that occurs in a small percentage of people with the skin condition psoriasis.

Raynaud's phenomenon: Exaggerated reduction in blood flow to the extremities (blanching) on exposure to cold, followed by excessive flushing (reddening).

Reactive arthritis: An inflammatory arthritis that develops within a few weeks of exposure to certain bacteria that infect the bowel or genito-urinary tract.

Rheumatoid arthritis: A chronic inflammatory arthritis that affects multiple joints, mostly in the hands and feet, usually symmetrically, and with the potential to erode the joints over many years.

Rheumatoid factor: An antibody found in the blood of 70 per cent of patients with rheumatoid arthritis — it can also be found in a small number of healthy people.

Scleroderma: An auto-immune vascular disease in which fibrous hardening occurs in the skin and internal organs such as the lungs.

Sjögren's syndrome: Inflammation of the tear and salivary glands causing dryness of the eyes and/or mouth.

Synovectomy: Surgical removal of the joint lining.

Synovial membrane: The thin layer inside a joint that gets inflamed in inflammatory arthritis.

Systemic lupus erythematosus: An auto-immune disease which can affect numerous organs and tissues, such as the joints, skin, blood cells, lungs, kidneys and brain.

Tendonitis: Inflammation of tendons and/or the linings of tendons.
Tendons: Fibrous bands that attach muscles to bones.

Uric acid crystals: Needle-shaped crystals of uric acid that deposit in and around joints, causing gout.

Vasodilators: Drugs that open up blood flow and are used in the treatment of Raynaud's phenomenon and high blood pressure.

Appendix 2:
Useful contacts

Websites

Every day more and more excellent information concerning arthritis is available through the internet. On the other hand there is much information that you'd do best to ignore. So how can you tell the good from the bad?

The best advice we can offer is to only visit sites that have been recommended by a responsible source and, then, only act on information once you've talked to your rheumatologist, doctor, rheumatology nurse or arthritis educator.

Here are the five sites we suggest visiting:

Arthritis New Zealand: <www.arthritis.org.nz>
New Zealand Rheumatology Association: <www.rheumatology.org.nz>
Arthritis Research Campaign: <www.arc.org.uk>
Arthritis Foundation (USA): <www.arthritis.org>
International League of Associations for Rheumatology: <www.ilar.org>

All these have links to other relevant and interesting sites that you can trust because they will have been scrutinised and approved by the original host site.

Arthritis New Zealand

There are a number of organisations throughout the country whose purpose is to offer aid and assistance to anyone who is affected by arthritis. Top of the list is Arthritis New Zealand, a not-for-profit organisation whose mission is to improve the health and wellbeing of people affected by arthritis.

Arthritis New Zealand has service centres throughout the country, each offering a range of services, which includes:

- Arthritis educators who provide individual and group support, education and advice — they will also refer you through to other agencies that may be of help
- Support groups — regular meetings and social events in many locations and for specialised needs, e.g. lupus support, craft groups, etc.
- Referral to exercise and hydrotherapy classes
- Educational resources, forums and seminars
- Information on self-management of chronic conditions
- Train the Leader Course, Living a Healthy Life — this course is available to organisations and trains leaders to run a six-week programme, which assists people to successfully self-manage chronic conditions
- A range of resources, aids and information

To find the service centre nearest you, check your local telephone directory under Arthritis New Zealand or contact the national office at:

Arthritis New Zealand, PO Box 10 020, Wellington
Phone: 04 472 1427
Freephone: 0800 663 463

Their website outlines the services they provide, information on different types of arthritis and ways to manage symptoms. It also has a forum where people have the opportunity to type in questions online, which will be answered by a rheumatologist. This website is well worth a visit at: <www.arthritis.org.nz>.

Your local District Health Board

You may be eligible for support through your local District Health Board (DHB) or the Ministry of Health by way of the Needs Assessment Service Coordination (NASC).

After carrying out an assessment of your needs, NASC will refer you to the appropriate service providers in your area; there is no charge for either the NASC assessment or the provider's service. You may be entitled to home help, assistance with personal care, home modification and equipment that will help you around the home.

NASCs are specially trained health professionals who are part of a nationally accredited organisation.

Contact points for NASC are as follows:

North Island

Auckland–Central Auckland: <www.adhb.govt.nz>
Service Name: NASC, Auckland DHB
Phone: 09 630 9943 ext 4735
Fax: 09 623 6461
Address: Greenlane Clinical Centre, Private Bag 92 024, Auckland

Auckland–North Shore & Rodney: <www.waitematadhb.govt.nz>
Service Name: NASC, Waitemata DHB
Phone: 09 486 8945 ext 2976
Fax: 09 486 8342
Address: North Shore Hospital, Private Bag 93 503, Takapuna, Auckland

Auckland–Waitakere: <www.waitematadhb.govt.nz>
Service Name: NASC, Waitemata DHB
Phone: 09 839 0000 ext 6303
Fax: 09 837 6664
Address: Waitakere Hospital, Private Bag 93 115, Henderson, Auckland

Auckland–Counties Manukau: <www.cmdhb.org.nz>
Service Name: NASC, Counties Manukau DHB
Phone: 09 276 0040
Fax: 09 276 0041
Address: NASC, Middlemore Hospital, PO Box 93 311, Otahuhu

Gisborne–Tairawhiti: <www.tdh.org.nz>
Service Name: Tairawhiti District Health, Community & Older People
Phone: 06 869 0500 ext 8507
Fax: 06 869 0554
Address: Gisborne Hospital, Private Bag 7001, Gisborne

Hamilton–Waikato: <www.waikatodhb.govt.nz>
Service Name: Disability Support Link — Health Waikato DHB

Phone: 07 839 1441 or 021 342 223
Fax: 07 839 1225
Address: Level 2, 73 Rostrevor St, PO Box 9210, Hamilton

Hokianga–Northland: <www.hokiangahealth.org.nz>
Service Name: Hauora Hokianga / Hokianga Health Enterprise Trust
Phone: 09 405 7709
Fax: 09 405 7329
Address: Hokianga Health Hospital, Rawene, PB, Kaikohe

Lower Hutt & Upper Hutt — Hutt Valley: <www.huttvalleydhb.org.nz>
Service Name: Sigma NASC
Phone: 04 570 1400
Fax: 04 570 1402
Address: Pilmuir House, Hutt Valley DHB, PO Box 44 151, Lower Hutt

Masterton–Wairarapa: <www.wairarapa.dhb.org.nz>
Service Name: FOCUS, Wairarapa DHB
Phone: 06 378 9660
Fax: 06 370 5029
Address: PO Box 58, Masterton

Napier–Hawke's Bay: <www.hawkesbaydhb.govt.nz>
Service Name: Bay Home Support, Hawke's Bay DHB
Phone: 06 870 7485
Fax: 06 870 7481
Address: 76 Wellesley Rd, PO Box 447, Napier

Northland Region: <www.nhl.co.nz>
Service Name: Community Assessment & Rehabilitation Services, Northland DHB
Phone: 09 430 4131
Fax: 09 430 4128
Address: Whangarei Area Hospital, PO Box 742, Whangarei

Palmerston North–Mid Central: <www.midcentral.co.nz>
Service Name: Supportlinks

Phone: 06 953 5800
Fax: 06 953 5822
Address: 60 Bennett St, PO Box 188, Palmerston North

Rotorua–Lakes: <www.lakesdhb.govt.nz>
Service Name: Support Net — Kupenga Hao Ite Ora, Pacific Health Ltd
Phone: 07 349 4213 or 0800 262 477
Fax: 07 349 3555
Address: 1143 Haupapa St, PO Box 1858, Rotorua

Taranaki: <www.tdhb.org.nz>
Service Name: Access Ability — Taranaki
Phone: 06 758 0700
Fax: 06 758 5201
Address: Level 2, Metro Plaza, 33 Devon St West, New Plymouth

Tauranga–Bay of Plenty: <www.bopdhb.govt.nz>
Service Name: Support Net — Kupenga Hao Ite Ora, Pacific Health Ltd
Phone: 07 571 0093
Fax: 07 571 0277
Address: 510 Cameron Rd, PO Box 2121, Tauranga

Waiheke Island–Auckland: <www.adhb.govt.nz>
Service Name: Waiheke Island Health Trust
Phone: 09 372 8893
Fax: 09 372 6787
Address: 5 Belgium St, Ostend, Waiheke Island

Wanganui: <www.wdhb.org.nz>
Service Name: Access Ability — Wanganui
Phone: 06 348 8411
Fax: 06 348 0166
Address: 126 Guyton St, Wanganui

Wellington–Capital & Coast: <www.ccdhb.org.nz>
Service Name: Links for Living, Capital Support, Capital Coast Health
Phone: 04 237 2570

Fax: 04 237 2571

Address: Level 3, Wrightson House, PO Box 50137, Porirua City

Whakatane–Bay of Plenty: <www.bopdhb.govt.nz>
Service Name: Support Net–Kupenga Hao Ite Ora, Pacific Health Ltd
Phone: 07 306 0986
Fax: 07 306 0987
Address: Stewart Street, PO Box 241, Whakatane

South Island

Canterbury Region: <www.cdhb.govt.nz>
Service Name: Older Persons Health, Canterbury DHB
Phone: 03 337 7765
Fax: 03 337 7720
Address: Princess Margaret Hospital, 2nd Floor, Heathcote Building, PO Box 800, Christchurch

Greymouth–West Coast: <www.westcoastdhb.org.nz>
Service Name: Coast Healthcare DHB, Needs Assessment
Phone: 768 0499 ext 2686
Fax: 768 2699
Address: Grey Base Hospital, PO Box 387, Greymouth

Nelson–Marlborough: <www.nmdhb.govt.nz>
Service Name: Support Works, Nelson–Marlborough DHB
Phone: 03 546 3980 or 0800 244 300
Fax: 03 546 3983
Address: 14 New St, Nelson

Otago Region: <www.otagodhb.govt.nz>
Service Name: Assessment & Support for Older People
Area Covered: Fairfield, Mosgiel, Port Chalmers, Otago peninsula, rural area south to Henly, west to Middlemarch, rural areas north to Waikouaiti and Palmerston
Phone: 03 476 6004 or 03 474 0999
Fax: 03 474 7026
Address: Dunedin Hospital, Ground Floor, PB 1921, Dunedin

Southland Region: <www.southlandhealth.co.nz>
Service Name: NASC for Older People's Health, Southland DHB
Phone: 03 214 5725 or 03 218 1949 ext 8028 or 0800 223 225
Fax: 03 214 7237
Address: Southland Hospital, PO Box 828, Invercargill

Timaru–South Canterbury: <www.scdhb.co.nz>
Service Name: NASC, South Canterbury DHB
Phone: 03 687 7120
Fax: 03 684 8819
Address: Cantec House, 24 George St, Level 5, PO Box 222, Timaru

Financial assistance

Financial assistance may be available through your local Work and Income New Zealand office (WINZ). There are a variety of benefits available and all have eligibility criteria.

If you want to apply for income support the first thing you should do is call WINZ on their freephone (0800 559 009) to arrange a meeting at their office nearest your home. The earlier you contact them the better, because usually they can't backdate payments.

When you call, they'll arrange a meeting and tell you what you need to bring with you. And remember you're always welcome to have someone with you for support. In most cases they'll tell you at your meeting if you qualify and how they can help.

Here is a list of some of the benefits that are available:

Invalids Benefit (IB): To receive an IB you must be aged 16 or over and be permanently and severely restricted in your capacity to work because of sickness, injury or disability.

Sickness Benefit: The Sickness Benefit provides income support for anyone who can't work due to sickness, injury, disability or pregnancy.

Disability Allowance (DA): This allowance reimburses people for ongoing regular costs that they incur because they have a disability. There is an income test and the amount of allowance paid depends on a person's costs.

Accommodation Supplement: An Accommodation Supplement is a non-taxable benefit that provides assistance towards your accommodation costs. You do not have to be receiving a benefit to qualify for an Accommodation Supplement.

Child Disability Allowance (CDA): This allowance is a fortnightly non-means-tested payment (it is a set weekly rate and is non-taxable) that can be made to the parent or guardian of a seriously disabled child who lives at home and requires constant care and attention. This allowance may also be available when the child lives in a home or hostel and the child's parent or guardian is required to contribute to the costs of maintaining them.

In some circumstances you may be eligible for help with your power and phone bills, and transport charges.

Community Services Card

You may be eligible for a Community Services Card, which would help you and your family with the costs of health care. Cards are issued by WINZ.

What does the card entitle you to?

You'll pay less on doctors' fees — each visit to your GP will be subsidised. The current subsidy (January 2006) is:

> Adult $15.00
>
> Child six years or over $20.00

If you have children under six, you'll automatically get a subsidy on doctors' fees, with or without a Community Services Card.

You will pay less for prescriptions. Everybody pays a 'government prescription charge' for prescription items that are subsidised by the government. Sometimes there is also a 'premium' or 'top up' to pay if the cost to manufacture the item is more than the government subsidy.

If you have a Community Services Card, all you'll pay is $3 for a subsidised prescription item, but you will still have to pay any premium. The amount of the prescription charge and the premium can change.

There are no government prescription charges on items for children under six, though there may still be a manufacturer's charge on some items which you'll have to pay.

The Community Services Card does not subsidise visits to private health professionals such as rheumatologists, physiotherapists, osteopaths, etc.

Remember, the freephone number for Work and Income is: 0800 559 009. They will put you in touch with your area office.

Their website at: <www.workandincome.govt.nz> carries a wealth of information.

Local and regional councils

If you can't drive and find it difficult to walk any distance your local council is likely to help you with some form of mobility allowance linked to either bus or taxi costs. If you're still driving, but find it difficult to walk, they're also likely to have a voucher scheme enabling you to park in the designated disabled car parking bays.

Your council may also offer reduced rates at swimming pools and gymnasiums and if you have a Community Services Card most council libraries will give you a discount if you take out music CDs, VCRs or DVDs.

For full information about all the services they offer, contact your local council.

Accident Compensation Corporation

In general, the Accident Compensation Corporation (ACC) is unable to assist with conditions that arise primarily from disease, unless that disease meets particular criteria, or is a personal injury caused by work-related circumstances.

If an ACC claimant has a pre-existing condition such as arthritis, and suffers a personal injury by accident which affects the arthritic site, then the personal injury caused by the accident may be accepted for cover although the pre-existing condition is not covered.

If the pre-existing condition has previously been accepted for cover by ACC (such as an earlier fracture site) then a worsened condition of that injury may be covered under the existing claim as a recurrence; for example, if arthritis has developed from the fracture, at the same site.

More information can be found on their website at: <www.acc.co.nz>. Click on 'Claims and Care/Entitlements'.

General health help

The Push Play programme aims to get New Zealanders off their sofas and into a more active life. It is organised by Sport and Recreation New Zealand (SPARC). You can find out more by contacting your local regional sports trust:

Freephone: 0800 ACTIVE (0800 228 483) and ask to speak to the Active Living Coordinator from your regional sports trust.

The Quit Group is a charitable trust formed by the Cancer Society, Te Hou Manawa Maori and the Health Sponsorship Council. It was set up to help New Zealanders give up smoking. One of the ways they help is by offering subsidised nicotine patches and gum, but if you have heart disease, are pregnant or are breast-feeding, you must talk to your doctor before using them.

Their address is:

PO Box 12 605, Thorndon, Wellington
Phone: 0800 778 778
Fax: 04 470 7632
Website: <ww.quit.org.nz>

Appendix 3:
Further resources

Inspirational reading material

Aisbett, B. *Living with it: A survivor's guide to panic attacks*, Angus & Robertson, an imprint of HarperCollins Publishers, Australia, 1993.

Ciurlionis, M. *A twist of fate: Tackling arthritis, New Zealanders share their stories*, Trio Books, Wellington, 2003.

Fisher, R. & Powers, M. *The knight in rusty armour*, Wilshire Book Company, California, 1989.

Grad, M. *The princess who believed in fairy tales: A story for modern times*, Wilshire Book Company, California, 1995.

General reading material

Britton, C., PhD. *Kids with Arthritis: A guide for families, Choices for families of children with arthritis*, United Kingdom, 2004.

Culling, C. *Arthritis Information and advice for New Zealanders*, GP Publications, Wellington, 1998.

Holden, T. *Talking about lupus: What to do and how to cope*, Piatkus Books, London, 2004.

Lorig, K., RN, DrPH & Fries, J., MD. *The Arthritis helpbook*, Perseus Books, Cambridge, Massachusetts, 2000.

Pitzele, S. K. *We are not alone: Learning to live with a chronic illness*, Workman Publishing, New York, 1986.

Appendix 4:

Medication

Note: Drugs whose names start with a small letter are generic; brand names always start with a capital letter.

There are a large number of medications your doctor can prescribe for you, not only to ease pain but also to relieve inflammation and keep your condition under control. Unfortunately, there's no single magic pill that can do it and you'll more than likely have to work with your doctor to find the combination of drugs that suits you best.

Medicines and risk

Almost all of the medical treatments that you'll be offered have the potential to cause side effects. This doesn't mean that they shouldn't be prescribed; arthritis has the potential to wreck peoples' lives and medication can make the difference between difficulty functioning and full participation in society. Medication can also minimise the damage caused by inflammatory arthritis. By monitoring your condition with regular clinic visits and blood tests any harmful side effects can be kept to an acceptable minimum.

When the risk of harm from arthritis is high and the risk of side effects is low, it makes sense to take medication. Don't be led astray by anecdotes from well-meaning friends and neighbours who may tell you horror stories that are often ill-informed. Don't be put off by the long list of possible (but usually extremely rare) side effects you may find on the internet or in the product package insert.

!! A medication will only be prescribed if the chance of benefit greatly outweighs the chance of harm.

Safe use of medication

There are a few simple guidelines to follow to ensure you are taking your medication correctly:

- Make sure you understand the medication that you're on and why it's been prescribed. If your doctor doesn't explain — ASK
- Tell your doctor if you're on any other non-arthritis medication, or if you're taking supplements
- Find out at what time of the day your medication should be taken and whether this should be before, after or with food
- If you forget to take your medication, DO NOT double-up. Consult your doctor or pharmacist
- Some medication can cause side effects — learn what these are; if you experience them and they persist, tell your doctor. There's almost always an alternative
- Tell your doctor of any unusual effects you experience
- Check if your medication prohibits drinking alcohol
- Keep your medication in its original containers
- Keep a list of your medicines and take it with you whenever you see your doctor
- Do not offer your medicines to others or take theirs
- If you visit your dentist tell them what medication you're on
- Make sure you take a supply of your medicines when going on holiday

!! Keep medicines away from children.

To get the right recipe for you, your doctor has five basic groups of drugs to choose from: analgesics, non-steroidal anti-inflammatory drugs (NSAIDs), corticosteroids, disease-modifying anti-rheumatic drugs (DMARDs) and biological agents.

Analgesics (pain relievers)

Paracetamol: This is a popular non-specific over-the-counter pain reliever available in New Zealand. A good starting medication for arthritis, it relieves many different types of pain and is well tolerated by the body.

Recommended dose: Usually 1000 mg (2 x 500 mg tablets) taken every four to six hours to a maximum of eight tablets per day.

Side effects: Generally safe at recommended doses, it can cause severe liver damage if taken in overdose.

Opiods: These are another form of pain reliever, and are related to morphine. They include: *codeine, tramadol* and *dextropropoxyphene.*

Side effects: The most common are drowsiness and constipation.

Non-steroidal anti-inflammatory drugs (NSAIDs)

These are not only particularly helpful in relieving inflammatory pain but will also help with non-inflammatory causes of pain.

Recommended dose: As these need to be taken under the supervision of your doctor, he will recommend the correct dose to suit your condition.

Side effects: The most well-known side effects are irritation and even ulceration of the stomach, which can lead to blood loss. Kidney problems can be made worse, but this medication rarely affects people with normal kidney function. You may experience side effects if you have high blood pressure.

Corticosteroids

Powerful inflammation relievers that are very useful in treating flares and sometimes given in low doses as a long-term treatment, corticosteroids can be injected or given in tablet form, usually as prednisone.

Recommended dose: As these need to be taken under the supervision of your doctor, he will suggest the correct dose to suit your condition.

Side effects: Most of the side effects of corticosteroids are dose-dependent, meaning the higher the dose, the more severe and the more rapid the onset of side effects. These include:

- In the short term — weight gain, mood changes, insomnia
- In the long term — obesity, thinning of the bones and skin (more of a problem in the elderly), unmasking of a tendency for diabetes, high blood pressure, cataracts

!! These drugs need to be used with caution in the elderly, in diabetics and in people with heart failure.

Such side effects may sound horrendous, but they are seldom seen if care is taken in prescribing the lowest possible doses and following up with careful monitoring. Injection of corticosteroid directly into the affected area maximises the effect and minimises the possibility of side effects.

Corticosteroids are a very useful treatment for severe inflammation and the fate of patients with inflammatory arthritis has been greatly improved thanks to these drugs.

Disease-modifying anti-rheumatic drugs (DMARDs)

Prescribed for chronic inflammatory arthritis, as with corticosteroids, DMARDs are not pain relievers as such but, by relieving inflammation, they relieve not only pain but also swelling and stiffness.

Whereas NSAIDs relieve the symptoms of inflammation (which persists), DMARDs reduce the underlying inflammation itself. This explains why DMARDs can prevent the damage caused by inflammation, whereas NSAIDs do not (because the inflammation persists).

Examples of DMARDs include: methotrexate (Methoblastin), sulphasalazine (Salazopyrine), hydroxychloroquine (Plaquenil), leflunomide (Arava), azathioprine (Imuran, Azamun), intramuscular gold (Myocrisin), and cyclosporine (Neoral).

This type of treatment takes a month or two to take effect, and, in all cases except hydroxychloroquine, requires monitoring with regular blood tests. For this reason this type of medication is reserved for patients who have:

- Chronic inflammatory symptoms
- Severe symptoms
- Risk of joint damage

Recommended dose: As these need to be taken under the supervision of your doctor, he will suggest the correct dose to suit your condition.

Side effects: These vary between the different drugs and may include: rash, nausea and blood-count or liver-function abnormalities. Rarely, more severe side effects may occur, but the benefits of these drugs for easing symptoms, preventing excessive corticosteroid use and preventing permanent damage outweigh the risks.

Biological agents

These are designer drugs that have been developed to target critical molecules in the inflammatory process. At present they are extremely expensive, with a year's treatment in New Zealand costing between $24,000 and $30,000. They are not publicly funded.

Index